"Nutrient Timing represents the next important nutrition concept in the twenty-first century and will teach readers how to optimize their exercise and recovery metabolism to better achieve their fitness and body-development goals. It is a must-read for anyone interested in physical fitness, performance, and health."

—William J. Kraemer, Ph.D.
Professor, University of Connecticut

"Drs. Ivy and Portman have made a major contribution to the field of sports nutrition. They've shown that consuming the right nutrients at the right time optimizes the adaptive response of skeletal muscle."

—Jose Antonio, Ph.D., C.S.C.S., F.A.C.S.M.
President, International Society of Sports Nutrition

"Drs. Ivy and Portman have written a classic. Their science filled book dispels old myths and should be mandatory reading for all strength athletes."

—Paul Goldberg, M.S., R.D., C.S.C.S.
Strength and Conditioning Coach, Colorado Avalanche

"The most important thing to add to your routine that will maximize your workouts is *Nutrient Timing*."

—Susan M. Kleiner, Ph.D., R.D., F.A.C.N., C.N.S.
Author of Power Eating

"Drs. Ivy and Portman take sports nutrition to a new level. Using some of the latest research they show how nutrients consumed at the appropriate time can work synergistically to stimulate enormous gains in muscle mass and strength— a must-read for the strength coach and athlete."

—Michael H. Stone, Ph.D.
Head, Sports Physiology, U.S. Olympic Committee

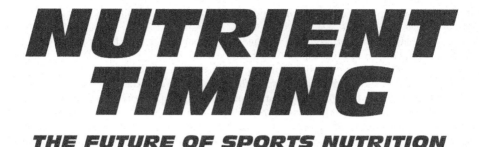

NUTRIENT TIMING

THE FUTURE OF SPORTS NUTRITION

John Ivy, Ph.D., & Robert Portman, Ph.D.

Foreword by William Kraemer, Ph.D.

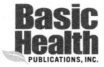

Basic Health
PUBLICATIONS, INC.

The information contained in this book is based upon the research and personal and professional experiences of the authors. It is not intended as a substitute for consulting with your physician or other healthcare provider. Any attempt to diagnose and treat an illness should be done under the direction of a healthcare professional.

The publisher does not advocate the use of any particular healthcare protocol but believes the information in this book should be available to the public. The publisher and authors are not responsible for any adverse effects or consequences resulting from the use of the suggestions, preparations, or procedures discussed in this book. Should the reader have any questions concerning the appropriateness of any procedures or preparation mentioned, the authors and the publisher strongly suggest consulting a professional healthcare advisor.

Basic Health Publications, Inc.
www.basichealthpub.com

Library of Congress Cataloging-in-Publication Data

Ivy, John.
   Nutrient timing : the future of sports nutrition / John Ivy and Robert Portman ; foreword by William Kraemer.
      p. cm.
   Includes bibliographical references and index.
   ISBN 978-1-59120-141-0 (Pbk.)
   ISBN 978-1-68162-760-1 (Hardcover)

   1. Athletes—Nutrition.   I. Portman, Robert.   II. Title.

   TX361.A8I98   2004
   613.2'024'796—dc22   2004000717

Editor: Carol Rosenberg
Typesetter/Book design: Gary A. Rosenberg
Cover design: Mikey Gudikunst

Contents

In Memory of

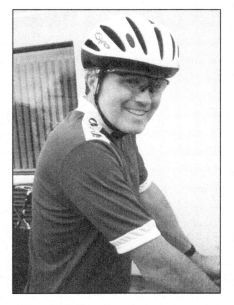

Dr. Ed Burke (1950–2002)

*Educator, inventor, scientist, coach, mentor, trainer,
author, fitness guru, missionary for sport,
and, most of all, a cherished friend*

Acknowledgments

We are grateful to the many people who have helped make this book possible. Joey Antonio, Jeff Stout, Matt Fitzgerald, and William Kraemer offered valuable suggestions and comments. Special thanks to John Berardi, whose practical observations are found in a number of chapters, and Susan Kleiner, who helped synthesize the science into an easy-to-follow daily nutrition program.

We would like to acknowledge Norman Goldfind at Basic Health Publications, who recognized the value of this information and encouraged us to write this book. Special gratitude to Carol Rosenberg, whose expertise and patience have shepherded this project to successful completion in spite of a very difficult time schedule. Additional thanks to Mina Rathbun for the medical illustrations, Nancy Martino for her creative suggestions for the cover, and Gary Rosenberg, whose design creativity has made this book come alive.

Most of all, we would like to thank the many researchers and athletes with whom we have been associated over the years, whose insights, experience, and studies represent the scientific underpinnings as well as the practical application of Nutrient Timing.

Finally, we would like to thank our wives, Jennifer and Susan, who have been so supportive of the time and effort necessary to complete this book.

Foreword

In the world of exercise and nutrition, a plethora of books have come out on a host of topics, but only a few will have a dramatic impact on the field. This is one of those books! It was written by two consummate scientists who have actually done the work in the laboratory to develop the theory and test the hypotheses that this book is based on. Therefore, different from so many of the books in the nutrition and exercise field that line the bookshelves in any bookstore, this book is the real thing based on scientific facts. Nutrient Timing represents the next important nutrition concept in the twenty-first century and will teach readers how to optimize their exercise and recovery metabolism to better achieve their fitness and body-development goals. It is a must-read for anyone interested in physical fitness, performance, and health.

This book provides readers with a well thought out structure so that they can actually develop a comprehensive understanding of what Nutrient Timing is all about. It is well written and provides the needed documentation to help athletes understand the reasoning behind the different elements of the program. Most important, it is easy to read, and this is accomplished by a very well thought out presentation style and topic structure. Finally, it is fun to read as the story of Nutrient Timing is so vividly portrayed and illustrated with graphs and stories about studies that one forgets it is a scientifically based book and not an exciting novel.

Implementing the concepts of Nutrient Timing will have a dramatic impact on the success of any exercise program, giving this book tremendous practical value. Whether one is a distance runner or weight trainer or any combination, the use of Nutrient Timing is vital in an athlete's ability to optimize exercise performance and, even more important, to promote the optimal recovery from the exercise stress of a workout. Thus, the practical benefits from reading this book are real and immense! It allows readers to understand the reasons why something needs to be done in specific order as well as how the body will adapt and respond. This book provides a step-by-step guide on how to implement and use the concept in a personalized exercise and nutrition program. One of the many interesting features of this book is the use of "Key Takeaways" at the end of each chapter, which underscore what readers should know and take away from their reading. Impacting the clarity and style of the book, the authors have carefully considered what readers must get out of a chapter before they move on. This book provides readers with the opportunity to reflect as they develop the needed understanding of the Nutrient Timing concept for use in their own exercise and nutrition program.

Finally, I am really excited about this book Nutrient Timing because it brings together in a most eloquent manner an important concept in the field of nutrition and exercise today. It allows readers to really understand the scientific basis of the concept. It takes them through an exciting and interesting development of the concept. It is easy to read and understand because the information is presented in a manner that allows readers to enjoy the learning experience as they become partners in developing this concept for their own practical use. It is a complete look at the concept with practical elements that will dramatically impact anyone's training program.

I hope that you will enjoy this book as much as I have and, after reading it, feel that you too now possess some powerful new tools that will help you optimize your workouts with better use of Nutrient Timing! Enjoy.

—William J. Kraemer, Ph.D.
Professor, University of Connecticut

Introduction

Nutrient Timing is a revolutionary new system of exercise nutrition that will allow you to build more strength and lean muscle mass in less time than ever before. Its methods are safe and natural, and can be used by anyone—from children to the elderly and from beginning exercisers to professional bodybuilders and power lifters. Nutrient Timing is not a commercial gimmick. Rather, it is the fruit of cutting-edge scientific insights into exercise metabolism, physiology, and nutrition.

The seeds of the Nutrient Timing revolution were planted twenty years ago. Before then, sports nutrition for muscle building and strength training was in the dark ages. It was based on unproven claims, myths, and practices that were not only useless but sometimes even dangerous. There was a feeling that nutrition could help increase muscle strength and lean body mass and stimulate muscle growth, but there wasn't much science to support it.

Hoping to correct this situation, exercise physiologists and nutritionists initiated research studies that measured the effect of increased protein consumption on muscle growth and strength. The results were dramatic. This was the beginning of a revolution in sports nutrition for strength athletes. Old ideas were quickly discarded and a new nutritional paradigm was established. The new paradigm challenged the recommended daily allowance (RDA) for essential nutrients. Protein intake was emphasized and carbohydrate intake de-emphasized. Athletes got results. Thus, "protein" has been the mantra among those involved in resistance training for the last fifteen years.

However, as strength athletes became more intelligent about nutrition and began adopting the new nutrition paradigm with good results, they began to notice what is called the "plateau phenomenon." This phenomenon is characterized by stagnation in muscle strength and growth. Even following the established recommended exercise and diet guidelines did not seem to prevent the plateau phenomenon from occurring.

Eager to tackle this problem, we, along with other colleagues, have become involved in groundbreaking sports-nutrition research. This research adds a new dimension to sports nutrition—the dimension of time. Until now, the strength athlete has focused entirely on *what* to eat. The latest research is providing powerful proof that *when* nutrients are consumed may be even more important. This emerging research on nutrition and how to activate natural anabolic (muscle-building) agents is again changing the way we look at building muscle. These findings form the underpinnings of the next revolution in sports nutrition—Nutrient Timing—which promises to help athletes break through plateaus and achieve higher levels of strength and power.

The easiest way to understand the principles of Nutrient Timing is to look at how the automobile fuel system evolved. In older cars, the primary fuel-delivery device was the carburetor. Older carburetors delivered a crude mixture of oxygen and gasoline to the pistons, which converted this mixture into the power that drives the car. If too much oxygen or gasoline was added to the carburetor, the engine stalled. Carburetors were the standard for almost 100 years, but eventually they gave way to fuel injectors. Fuel injectors are far more efficient in converting oxygen and gas into maximum energy because the mixture is delivered at precisely the time when the piston needs it. Newer cars even have a computer that drives the fuel injectors, making the timing of the delivery of fuel even more precise. As a result, today's cars get better performance out of the same tank of gas.

That's what Nutrient Timing is all about. Until now, strength athletes have used an old carburetor approach to generate muscle growth and energy. The only improvement has been in the type of fuel. We know that certain types of protein are "higher octane" and give better results. But the high-octane protein is still being delivered with imprecise timing by an old "carburetor." By following the principles of Nutrient Timing, you'll be able to deliver the precise amounts of protein and other necessary nutrients at precisely the right time to maximize muscle growth.

Some of the leading sports scientists from the fields of nutrition, exercise physiology, and molecular biology have contributed to these findings. Nutrient Timing is a program built on science. This book includes references to many of the scientific studies related to Nutrient Timing and also provides an extensive bibliography so that you can review the studies yourself, if you wish.

The exciting new science of Nutrient Timing will enable you to achieve more dramatic results in muscle growth and strength than you ever thought possible. Nutrient Timing will enable you to minimize muscle damage and soreness after a hard workout, and your "plateau phenomenon" will become just a bad memory. By applying the principles of Nutrient Timing, you can actually sculpt a better body with more lean muscle mass, less fat, and more power without changing your exercise program or even your total caloric intake.

Nutrient Timing is, above all, a practical program. The information in this book will change the way you look at nutrition and, more important, change the results you get from your hard time in the gym. We'll show you specifically how to apply the latest findings to change the way your body builds muscle, burns fat, and stores energy for the next workout.

As scientists, we are excited about these findings. As athletes, we are applying them to our own programs and have experienced results firsthand. Nutrient Timing is the future of sports nutrition. Read on to learn how to make it work for you.

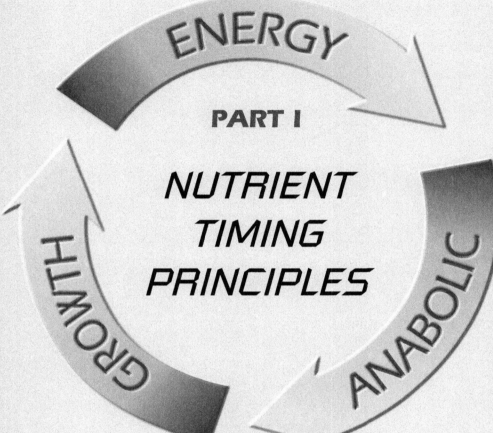

ENERGY

GROWTH

ANABOLIC

PART I

NUTRIENT TIMING PRINCIPLES

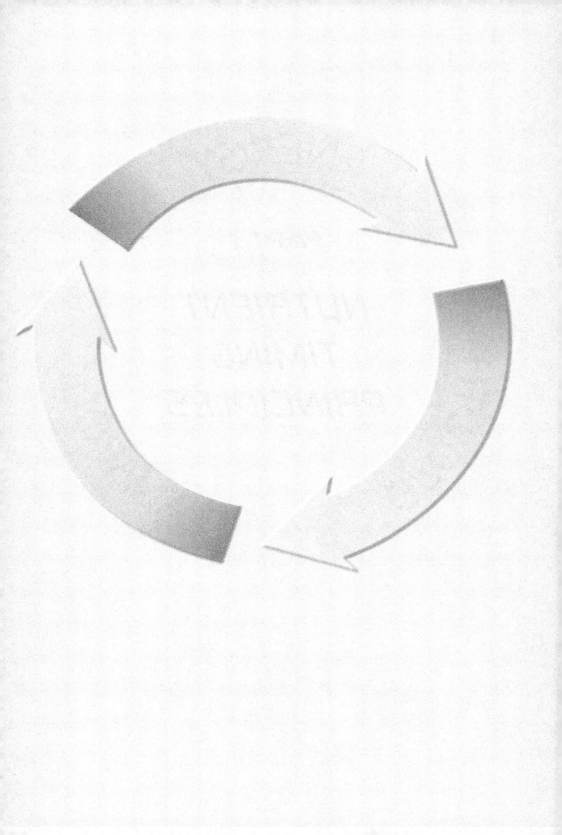

Nutrient Timing

During a muscle's twenty-four-hour growth cycle, there are periods when the muscle is actively involved in producing energy, periods when it is recovering, and periods when it is growing. For the metabolic machinery of the muscle to function at its best during each of these periods, the appropriate amounts and types of nutrients must be consumed at the appropriate times.

Depending on its metabolic needs at any given time, the muscle machinery can be directed to produce and replenish muscle glycogen (the stored form of glucose) or synthesize muscle protein. Each of these operations requires different types of nutrients, and if you're able to deliver the right nutrient mixture to the muscles at the right time, you can greatly enhance recovery from exercise and improve muscle growth, strength, and power.

To understand why Nutrient Timing is such a revolutionary concept, we must first take a look at sports nutrition over the past twenty years. The focus of sports nutrition has been on the types of nutrients that are best for the strength athlete. It was quickly recognized that strength athletes need more protein than is recommended for the average person and that an increased consumption of protein could improve muscle development.

This has led to a "bulk nutrition" mentality. If protein is good, then more protein must be better. Unfortunately, you can consume the protein of an entire cow, but if your muscles are not receptive at that particular time, the protein will be wasted. And, in fact, the evidence indicates that very few strength athletes fail to get enough protein to support muscle growth. Then why do so many athletes plateau in their training? The answer lies in *when* nutrients are consumed, which is what Nutrient Timing is all about. By consuming the same amount of nutrients, but keying your consumption to the three phases of muscle growth discussed below, you will be able to avoid the plateau effect and achieve far greater gains in muscle strength and muscle mass.

THE THREE PHASES OF THE NUTRIENT TIMING SYSTEM (NTS)

There are three phases of the Nutrient Timing System: the Energy Phase, the Anabolic Phase, and the Growth Phase.

The Energy Phase

The Energy Phase coincides with your workout. The primary metabolic objective of the muscle during this phase is to release sufficient energy to drive muscle contraction. Most athletes recognize the importance of consuming carbohydrates during exercise both to prevent depletion of muscle glycogen stores, which helps extend endurance, and to maintain blood glucose levels, which helps delay fatigue. Nutrient Timing, however, entails more than just consuming carbohydrates during exercise. Research has shown that when you consume carbohydrates with protein, specific amino acids, and vitamins, you will be able to spare muscle glycogen and achieve greater muscular endurance, blunt the rise in the catabolic hormone cortisol (thereby reducing muscle damage), and help prepare your muscle enzymes for a faster recovery following your workout.

The Anabolic Phase

The Anabolic Phase is the forty-five-minute window following a workout in which your muscle machinery, in the presence of the right combination of nutrients, initiates the repair of damaged muscle protein and replenishes muscle glycogen stores. Immediately after exercise, muscle cells are extremely sensitive to the anabolic effects of the hormone insulin. This sensitivity, however, declines rapidly, as shown in Figure 1.1, and, after several hours, muscle cells even become insulin resistant. Insulin resistance is a condition that dramatically slows muscle glycogen recovery, repair of existing muscle, and synthesis of new muscle.

As you read this book, you will come to understand why consumption of carbohydrates during this time period is so important for driving muscle glycogen recovery and muscle tissue repair and synthesis. You'll also learn why protein consumed without carbohydrate is far less efficient during the Anabolic Phase. Moreover, you'll learn why specific antioxidants such as vitamins C and E and amino acids can speed muscle recovery.

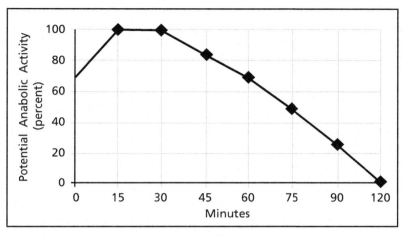

Figure 1.1. Closing of Metabolic Window
Without nutrient intervention, the metabolic window begins to close within forty-five minutes following exercise.

The Growth Phase

The Growth Phase extends from the end of the Anabolic Phase to the beginning of the next workout. It is the time when the muscle enzymes are involved in increasing the number of contractile proteins and the size of muscle fibers, as well as in helping the muscle fully replenish muscle glycogen depleted during the Energy Phase. During the Growth Phase, consumption of carbohydrate and protein is essential to maintain optimal muscle growth. The latest research shows that a high intake of protein can be of significant benefit to the strength athlete if protein is consumed at the correct time. By following the Nutrient Timing System, you'll be able to maintain a high anabolic state and restore muscle glycogen, repair muscle tissue damage, and synthesize new muscle.

IMPORTANT CONCEPTS IN THE NUTRIENT TIMING SYSTEM

The Nutrient Timing System is going to challenge much of what you've been taught to believe about exercise nutrition. For the past twenty years, nutritionists, exercise physiologists, and strength athletes have painted nutrients in black-and-white terms: "Sugar is bad and protein is good." These generalized prejudices may be useful in building an overall healthy diet, but they often don't take into account the metabolic realities of muscle cells during and after exercise.

Following are three true statements that most strength athletes would find pretty hard to believe. They illustrate important concepts in the Nutrient Timing System.

"A low-quality protein can be more effective in stimulating protein synthesis than a high-quality protein."

Everything that you have heard or read would suggest that the above statement is false. The shelves of health food stores are filled with products proclaiming their superiority because they contain a better-quality protein. However, the effectiveness of any protein product is largely dependent on *when* you take it.

Muscles can modify their metabolic activity in response to changing needs and various stimuli at any given instant. This is called "metabolic sensitivity." A good example is the effect of the hormone insulin. If insulin is stimulated when you are not exercising, it can cause a conversion of carbohydrate into fat, which is the last thing a strength athlete needs. However, in the forty-five minutes after a workout (the Anabolic Phase), the metabolic machinery of the muscle is extremely sensitive to insulin. Insulin has been shown to drive the rebuilding, or anabolic activity, of the muscle. Nutrients consumed during this postexercise "metabolic window" are much more effective than those consumed later, when the muscle becomes insulin resistant.

Let's look at our shocking but true statement in the light of Nutrient Timing. Consuming a poor-quality protein, such as corn, during the forty-five-minute postexercise metabolic window will actually result in greater protein synthesis than consuming a high-quality protein, such as whey protein isolate, two hours later. And the difference is not small. The high-quality protein consumed two hours later may result in 85 percent less protein synthesis compared with the corn protein taken immediately after the workout. In Chapter 5, you will find out why.

"Sugar can stimulate protein synthesis."

For strength athletes, "sugar," or carbohydrate, is the poster boy for bad nutrition. Nutrition articles in bodybuilding and strength-training publications routinely discuss the negative effects of carbohydrates. Much of what they say is true—up to a point. Unfortunately, your muscle cells do not read articles appearing in the popular press. This brings us to the second essential concept of Nutrient Timing. It's called "nutrient activation."

Your muscle cells never rely on a single nutrient. Rather, muscle metabolism is a tightly scripted symphony involving fat, carbohydrate, protein, vitamins, minerals, and water. The proportions of nutrients consumed can significantly affect the degree to which you are able to achieve the results you are seeking. Consuming too much carbohydrate may result in increased body fat. Consuming too much protein or consuming it at the wrong time may produce no benefit except to the manufacturers of protein powders.

An excellent example of nutrient activation is the addition of simple (high-glycemic) sugars to protein. Studies have shown that a high-glycemic carbohydrate/protein supplement can dramatically enhance protein synthesis. In fact, in one study, a high-glycemic carbohydrate/protein drink was 38 percent more effective in stimulating protein synthesis than a conventional protein drink.

The reason for this effect is that the high-glycemic carbohydrates can serve as nutrient activators. Consuming high-glycemic carbohydrates following exercise stimulates insulin, one of the most important regulators of protein synthesis following exercise. When insulin is stimulated in the presence of protein, the result is greater synthesis of new protein. In other words, carbohydrates prime the protein pump by first stimulating insulin. A complex carbohydrate is less effective because it is a weaker stimulator of insulin.

By now you may be thinking that this book is about the benefits of carbohydrates. It is not. But there are certain times—namely during and immediately following workouts—when the addition of simple carbohydrates can have dramatic effects on the muscle cells' anabolic processes, which can lead to greater increases in muscle strength and endurance.

"Sugar is more effective than protein in preventing protein degradation in the muscle."

The third important concept in the Nutrient Timing System is "nutrient optimization." The consumption of certain nutrients at specific times not only can help the muscle recover faster, but can also shift the metabolic machinery from a catabolic state into an anabolic one. Following strenuous exercise, there is a significant increase in blood cortisol levels. Cortisol is the enemy of strength athletes because it breaks down muscle protein; however, its release is a normal part of the body's response to the stress of exercise. By consuming carbohydrates during exercise, you can reduce the cortisol response and thereby lessen protein breakdown. Consumption of high-glycemic sugars increases blood insulin levels. Among its many effects, insulin prevents protein degradation. Thus, by increasing insulin levels postexercise in the presence of other essential nutrients such as protein, you can turn off the muscle's catabolic switch and turn on its anabolic one.

You may still be skeptical. However, we encourage you to reserve final judgment until you've read more about the Nutrient Timing System. We will challenge some of your long-held beliefs and introduce you to many new ideas about exercise and nutrition. You'll find that the bulk theory of protein consumption gives you a false sense of accomplishment and may even hinder muscle development. You'll learn about the critical metabolic window during which you have an opportunity to double or triple protein synthesis. You'll learn how carbohydrates can increase blood flow to your muscles, and you'll find out why two small helpings of protein may be more effective than a single large helping. Nutrient Timing can also show you how to reduce your susceptibility to colds and infection.

Finally, you will soon realize that the Nutrient Timing System is a simple one. You won't have to walk around with a stopwatch timing every meal to the last millisecond. All you'll have to do is recognize that there are critical times during and after exercise to stimulate the muscle's natural anabolic agents. Best of all, you'll see the results almost immediately.

Table 1.1 explains when the three Nutrient Timing phases fall in relation to your daily workout and the benefits of consuming the right combination of nutrients within each phase. Chapters 4, 5, and 6 describe the metabolic processes that take place in the three phases of your muscles' growth cycle and why nutrient intervention can play a critical role. And in Chapters 7 and 8, we show you how to easily incorporate the Nutrient Timing System into your own training program.

TABLE 1.1. Nutrient Timing System (NTS) Phases and Goals

NTS Phase	Time	What NTS Can Do for You
ENERGY	10 minutes prior to and during a workout	Increase nutrient delivery to muscles and spare muscle glycogen and protein
		Limit immune system suppression
		Minimize muscle damage
		Set the nutritional stage for a faster recovery following your workout
ANABOLIC	Within 45 minutes after a workout	Shift metabolic machinery from a catabolic state to an anabolic state
		Speed the elimination of metabolic wastes by increasing muscle blood flow
		Replenish muscle glycogen stores
		Initiate tissue repair and set the stage for muscle growth
		Reduce muscle damage and bolster the immune system
GROWTH	**Rapid Segment** The first 4 hours after a workout	Maintain increased insulin sensitivity
		Maintain the anabolic state
	Sustained Segment The next 16–18 hours after a workout	Maintain positive nitrogen balance and stimulate protein synthesis
		Promote protein turnover and muscle development

KEY TAKEAWAYS

- During a muscle's twenty-four-hour growth cycle, it is uniquely sensitive to specific nutrients at different times.

- The Nutrient Timing System divides the muscles' twenty-four-hour growth cycle into three phases: Energy Phase (your workout), Anabolic Phase (the first forty-five minutes after your workout), and Growth Phase (the rest of the day).

- If you deliver the right nutrient mixture to the muscles at the right time, you can improve muscle growth, strength, and power.

- Metabolic sensitivity is the inherent property of muscles to modify their function depending on the needs and nutrients available.

- Nutrient activation is the combined action of different nutrients to produce a synergistic effect.

- Nutrient optimization is the shifting of muscle from a catabolic state to an anabolic state by making available key nutrients at the appropriate time.

Muscle Energy Systems and Fuel Utilization

Exercise and nutrition have equal roles in relation to muscle development. Intense resistance exercise is required to stimulate muscle tissue remodeling and to increase muscle protein levels and other physiological adaptations that add up to bigger, stronger muscles. Nutrition is needed both to fuel workouts so that they can be more intense and stimulate more pronounced adaptations and to provide the raw materials for those adaptations that occur between workouts.

In order to best understand the NTS system, you need a basic understanding of the relationship between nutrition and energy production, on the one hand, and between nutrition and recovery, on the other hand. In this chapter, we will focus on how and where muscles derive their energy. If you would like more detailed information on muscle structure, function, and how to optimize muscle growth through training, please refer to Chapter 12.

ATP—THE ENERGY CURRENCY OF THE MUSCLE CELL

Muscle contraction requires a precise amount and appropriate timing of energy release from fuel stored in the muscle. When the muscle cell receives the signal from the brain to contract, energy stored in the form of adenosine triphosphate (ATP) is converted into the energy to drive contraction. This requires that a phosphate molecule be separated from ATP, forming adenosine diphosphate (ADP) and inorganic phosphate (Pi). ATP is the only source of energy that can drive muscle contraction. However, there is only enough ATP stored in the muscle to support a maximal effort for a few seconds. Therefore, ATP must be continually replenished or muscle contraction will stop.

To maintain ATP levels during contraction, the muscle relies on both anaerobic (without oxygen) and aerobic (with oxygen) energy systems as seen in Figure 2.1. The proportion of energy provided by these systems is intensity-related. The higher the intensity of contraction, the greater the reliance on the anaerobic energy system. The lower the intensity, the greater the reliance on the aerobic energy system. If you are doing six sets of squats, you will rely on your anaerobic energy system to produce ATP because squats are high-intensity, explosive movements. But if you are planning to jog a mile, you will rely on your aerobic system to produce ATP.

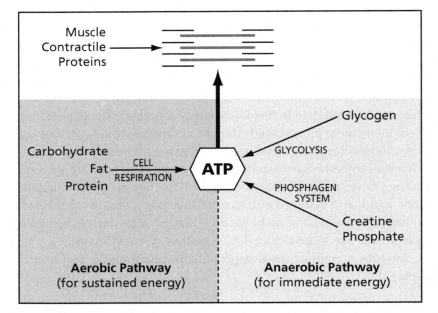

Figure 2.1. Muscle Energy Systems
ATP is the only molecule that drives muscle contraction. Since the amount of ATP in the muscle is very limited (enough for only two to three seconds of intense muscle activity), it must be continuously supplied through both anaerobic and aerobic pathways. There are two anaerobic pathways: the phosphagen and glycolytic pathways. These pathways provide immediate ATP but in limited amounts and are critical for high-intensity, short-duration exercise. The aerobic pathway is necessary for sustained energy. It is far more efficient in producing ATP than the anaerobic pathways, but cannot produce ATP as rapidly. The aerobic pathway provides energy for low- to moderate-intensity exercise of longer duration by using carbohydrates, fat, and even protein as fuel.

ANAEROBIC ENERGY SYSTEM

The anaerobic replenishment of ATP can occur either by the breakdown of creatine phosphate (CP), another high-energy compound stored in muscle like ATP, or by glycolysis.

Phosphagen System

Because ATP and CP are high-energy phosphate compounds, they are referred to as phosphagens, and the energy system in which these compounds are used for the liberation of energy for muscle contraction is referred to as the phosphagen system. CP is the immediate supplier of energy for the formation of ATP. As CP is broken down to creatine and Pi, it releases energy for the rapid replenishment of ATP. There is a sufficient amount of CP stored in the muscle to support a maximal effort for eight to twelve seconds. Without this system, fast, powerful movements such as sprinting could not be performed.

Glycolysis

A second anaerobic system in which ATP is produced is glycolysis. Glycolysis generates ATP by the breakdown of carbohydrate stored in the muscle in the form of glycogen and blood glucose. Glycolysis cannot produce ATP as fast as the breakdown of CP, but it is still considerably faster than aerobic metabolism. Unfortunately, glycolysis is a relatively inefficient means of producing ATP and one of its byproducts, lactic acid, if produced in high concentrations, will interfere with muscle contraction and adversely affect performance. However, glycolysis, like the phosphagen system, is extremely important at the onset of exercise, when oxygen availability is limited and when the energy demand exceeds the energy-producing capability of the aerobic energy system.

AEROBIC ENERGY SYSTEM

In order for the muscles to continuously produce the force needed during long-term physical activity, they must have a steady supply of energy. In the presence of oxygen, the muscle is able to break down carbohydrate, fat, and, when needed, protein to generate ATP. Aerobic metabolism, or "cellular respiration," is a very efficient way of generating energy for muscle contraction. However, there is a trade-off for this increased efficiency, which is an energy production slower than that of the anaerobic energy systems. Aerobic energy production occurs in small organelles within the muscle fiber called "mitochondria." The mitochondria are like small energy-producing factories, which convert the energy stored in carbohydrate and fat into ATP. The more mitochondria in a muscle, the greater the muscle's potential for aerobic energy production.

Carbohydrate as a Fuel Source

The carbohydrate that is used during aerobic metabolism comes from the muscle glycogen stores and blood glucose. Glycogen is the form in which carbohydrate is stored in the body. In an average-size man, about 525 grams of glycogen are stored in the muscle with another 25 grams of glucose in the blood. The liver stores an additional 100 grams of glycogen, which can be broken down to glucose and released into the blood to maintain blood glucose as it is being used by the tissues of the body. The amount of energy stored as carbohydrate in the body is about 2,600 calories, of which 80 percent or 2,000 calories can be used. This is enough energy for about two hours of moderate exercise.

Figure 2.2 summarizes the energy characteristics of the different metabolic pathways.

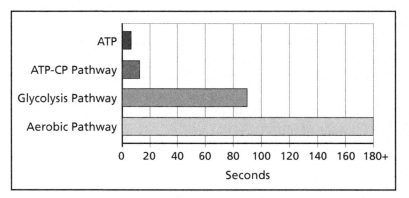

Figure 2.2. Relative Duration of Exercise Performance When Maximizing Energy Utilization from the Different Metabolic Pathways

Fat as a Fuel Source

Fat is the body's most concentrated fuel source. Unlike carbohydrate stores in your body, fat stores can fuel hours of exercise without running out. In fact, a 200-pound man with 15 percent body fat has stored about

130,000 calories of energy. This is enough energy to run from Washington, D.C., to Miami. However, because the majority of fat is stored in adipose tissue, it is not readily available for fueling the muscles. In order to be used as fuel, it must first be broken down into fatty acids, transported from the adipose tissue to the muscle by the circulatory system, and transported across the plasma membrane of the muscle and then into the mitochondria. Only in the mitochondria can fatty acids be broken down to provide the energy for ATP synthesis. This is not a very fast process and therefore energy from fatty acids can be used only during low- to moderate-intensity exercise.

Protein as a Fuel Source

The use of protein for ATP production occurs when carbohydrate stores are low. Proteins are made up of amino acids. Of the twenty amino acids that the body uses to make protein, eleven are designated as "nonessential" because they can be produced by the body from other amino acids and do not need to be obtained from the diet. The other nine are essential amino acids, which the body cannot synthesize. All the essential amino acids must be present in order for the body to build or repair muscle. During exercise, when the glycogen stores of the liver and muscles are starting to become depleted, muscle proteins are broken down into amino acids and released into the blood. The amino acids are then carried to the liver and converted into glucose by a process known as gluconeogenesis. Once converted to glucose by the liver, the glucose is released back into the blood to help maintain the blood glucose level and to provide glucose for the active muscles.

SUMMARY

The muscle cell only contains enough ATP to support muscle contraction for a few seconds. Therefore, in order to produce sufficient amounts of ATP to drive contraction the muscle relies on several different energy systems. In general, these systems can be characterized by the exercise duration and intensity that they can support. The anaerobic systems, which include the phosphagen system and glycolysis, can provide ATP rapidly but for only short periods of time. The aerobic system is more efficient in generating ATP but it cannot respond as fast as the anaerobic system. The aerobic system provides the energy necessary to drive muscle contraction for extended periods of time.

KEY TAKEAWAYS

- ATP is the only energy source that can be directly used for muscle contraction.

- The anaerobic replenishment of ATP during muscle contraction can occur by the breakdown of CP and by glycolysis.

- The anaerobic replenishment of ATP is rapid but very inefficient.

- The anaerobic energy system is the predominant supplier of ATP during high-intensity exercise because of the rapid turnover of ATP.

- The aerobic energy system resides in the mitochondria of the muscle cell and requires oxygen for ATP production.

- The aerobic energy system can use carbohydrates, fats, and protein to replenish ATP.

- Using the aerobic energy system is an efficient way of replenishing ATP, but it is much slower than the anaerobic system.

- The aerobic energy system is the predominant supplier of ATP during low- to moderate-intensity exercise.

The Influence of Hormones on Muscle Growth and Development

Every athlete who does resistance exercise knows at least a little bit about hormones. They are the agents that drive muscle development. In general, athletes classify hormones as good (anabolic) or bad (catabolic). But this is too simplistic. Even the so-called "bad" hormones are essential because they break down nutrients that provide the energy to drive muscle contraction. Even the "good" ones often stimulate reactions, such as increased fat deposition, that are not considered beneficial to the strength athlete.

Hormones are chemical messengers. In response to certain stimuli, they are released from one organ and travel via the bloodstream to another (the target organ), where they initiate a specific cell reaction. Both catabolic and anabolic hormones are important for resistance training. Anabolic hormones stimulate rebuilding and repair reactions in the muscle. Catabolic hormones stimulate the breakdown of carbohydrate, fat, and even protein for energy.

The Nutrient Timing System focuses on stimulating the release of anabolic hormones to maximize muscle growth and development.

Hormones are released in response to three stimuli: other hormones, stimulation of nerve fibers (which is what you would expect during exercise), and also changes in the levels of certain nutrients in the blood. Using the principles of Nutrient Timing, you will learn how to turn on the anabolic hormones, and, at the same time, turn off the catabolic ones to maximize muscle growth and development.

Table 3.1 on the next page summarizes the effects of the catabolic and anabolic hormones.

TABLE 3.1. The Metabolic Effects of the Catabolic and Anabolic Hormones			
Catabolic Hormones	**Effect**	**Anabolic Hormones**	**Effect**
Glucagon	Stimulates fat and liver glycogen breakdown and gluconeogenesis	Testosterone	Blocks cortisol and stimulates protein synthesis
Epinephrine	Stimulates fat, liver, and muscle glycogen breakdown	Growth hormone	Stimulates bone and cartilage growth and protein synthesis
Norepinephrine	Stimulates fat and liver glycogen breakdown	IGF-I	Stimulates growth of bone, cartilage, and muscle
Cortisol	Stimulates fat, liver glycogen, and muscle protein breakdown	Insulin	Multiple effects on muscle protein synthesis, protein degradation, and glycogen replenishment

CATABOLIC HORMONES

The four major catabolic hormones are glucagon, epinephrine, norepinephrine, and cortisol. They break down fuel stores such as fat and glycogen, and, in the case of cortisol, protein.

Glucagon

Glucagon is released from the pancreas. Glucagon is often called an "insulin antagonist." Insulin is stimulated by high blood glucose. Insulin shuttles glucose into the muscle, thereby lowering the blood glucose level. Glucagon, on the other hand, is released in the presence of low blood glucose. Its primary function is to raise the blood glucose concentration by increasing the release of glucose from the liver and by activating gluconeogenesis, the conversion of amino acids and other small compounds such as lactic acid to glucose. Additionally, glucagon increases the breakdown of fat. During exercise, glucagon is usually elevated.

Epinephrine (Adrenaline) and Norepinephrine (Noradrenaline)

Epinephrine is released from the adrenal glands in response to low levels of blood glucose as well as by the stimulation of resistance exercise. Norepinephrine is primarily released from nerve endings in blood vessels in response to exercise—the higher the intensity, the greater the increase.

Both hormones promote the breakdown of liver glycogen to glucose and its release into the blood, increase the breakdown of fat, and increase blood flow to the muscle. Epinephrine also stimulates muscle glycogen breakdown. Epinephrine and norepinephrine also have multiple physiological effects, including increasing respiration and heart rate. Both hormones are elevated during exercise as the body attempts to get more blood to the working muscles and to increase the breakdown of glycogen and fat for energy.

Cortisol

Cortisol is well known by strength athletes. This hormone is released from the adrenal glands when blood glucose is low and during very intense exercise such as weightlifting. Cortisol's major function is to generate fuel for working muscles. During exercise, your muscles use a metabolic priority system for generation of energy. This is particularly true during aerobic exercise. First, carbohydrate is used, then fat, and finally protein. Because of the tremendous stress that resistance training places on the muscles, the metabolic priority system gets ignored. When cortisol is released, it causes a breakdown of protein, carbohydrate, and fat and an increase in plasma amino acids, specifically glutamine and the branched-chain amino acids (BCAAs).

Elevated cortisol levels have enormous implications for strength athletes. The harder the workout is, the greater the cortisol release, and the greater the resulting protein degradation. Cortisol is the reason that many strength athletes reach a plateau. The anabolic benefits of exercise can actually be negated by the catabolic effect of cortisol.

ANABOLIC HORMONES

Anabolic hormones are involved in the rebuilding and replenishment processes of the muscle cell. The anabolic hormones include testosterone, growth hormone, IGF-1, and insulin.

Testosterone

Testosterone is a powerful anabolic hormone that is released from the testes in males and from the ovaries and adrenal glands in females. The release of testosterone is controlled by another hormone, luteinizing hormone (LH). LH is secreted from the pituitary, a gland found at the base of the brain. Testosterone has a number of effects, which are classified as either androgenic or anabolic. The androgenic effects include changes in sex organs and voice pitch and increased hair growth on the face and body, and psychological effects such as increased aggressiveness. The anabolic effects of testosterone include accelerated growth of muscle, bone, and red blood cells.

It is believed that testosterone, by blocking cortisol, has an anti-catabolic effect. Through this action, testosterone may speed muscle recovery. Athletes who use testosterone and its derivatives, including anabolic steroids, claim that these drugs help them train harder and recover faster. These effects tend to be short-lived, however. One reason is that when cortisol release is blocked for a period of time, higher levels of cortisol are produced thereafter. Thus, when an athlete stops taking an anabolic steroid such as testosterone, the catabolic effects of cortisol are enhanced and muscle strength and size are lost at a rapid rate.

Testosterone also has an effect on net protein synthesis. Researchers have shown that following five days of testosterone injections, there was a twofold increase in protein synthesis, whereas protein breakdown was unchanged. In a longer trial, over six months it appeared that the primary effect of testosterone was a decrease in protein breakdown. Taken together, these results suggest that the specific effects of testosterone on protein synthesis may be a function of the duration of treatment.

During exercise, there is a slight elevation in testosterone. This elevation is transitory, and most researchers believe it does not play an important role in the muscle's postexercise anabolic activities.

Growth Hormone

Growth hormone is released from the pituitary, and its release is controlled by a number of factors. Growth hormone stimulates muscle growth, increases the breakdown of fat, and inhibits carbohydrate metabolism. The role of growth hormone in exercise is not understood. There is a transient elevation that drops following exercise. Studies in endurance athletes show a minimal rise in blood levels of growth hormone during exercise when compared with untrained individuals.

IGF-1

IGF-1 stands for insulin-like growth factor. It is released from a variety of organs, including the pituitary gland, the muscles, and the liver. The primary effect of IGF-1 is stimulation of protein synthesis in bone, cartilage, and muscle. IGF-1 release is controlled by the intensity of muscle contractions. During exercise, there is a transient increase that falls to baseline following exercise.

Insulin

Insulin may be the most misunderstood hormone among strength athletes because of its association with carbohydrate. High levels of insulin combined with high carbohydrate intake have been shown to increase fat synthesis and decrease fat breakdown. Chronic elevation of blood insulin levels maintained over many years with the resulting accumulation of body fat is associated with type II (adult-onset) diabetes.

However, while it's true that high levels of insulin promote fat synthesis, they do not necessarily do so to the same degree in all circumstances. Insulin is just as effective in promoting carbohydrate fuel storage and muscle protein synthesis. The degree to which insulin promotes fat storage, carbohydrate storage, or protein synthesis at any given time depends on certain aspects of the individual's body state. Perhaps the most important factor is the relative degree of insulin sensitivity in fat cells versus muscle cells: the more insulin sensitive the fat cells are at a given time, the more insulin will act to promote fat storage; the more insulin sensitive the muscle cells are, the more insulin will act to promote muscle glycogen storage and protein synthesis.

Muscle cells are especially insulin sensitive after exercise. If glucose and amino acids are made available at this time, insulin will help synthesize muscle proteins and muscle glycogen at a very rapid rate, and very little fat will be synthesized and stored in adipose (fat) tissue.

Lifestyle factors can increase the insulin sensitivity of the muscle cells and thereby create a body that is generally disposed to build muscle proteins and less disposed to store body fat. Exercise and a moderate-carbohydrate diet that is rich in fiber can increase muscle insulin sensitivity. Alternatively, a low-carbohydrate, high-fat diet can decrease insulin sensitivity, which, as you will soon see, can have negative effects on muscle mass and strength.

Because of its many actions, insulin has earned the title "anabolic regulator of the muscle." In fact, insulin may be the most important hormone to increase muscle strength and mass. Insulin is also at the heart of the Nutrient Timing System.

Insulin is released from the pancreas usually in response to high levels of blood glucose. Most people are familiar with the fact that insulin increases the transport of glucose into the muscle cell, but insulin plays many more roles, as you will quickly learn.

INSULIN INCREASES PROTEIN SYNTHESIS

Insulin has a number of actions that increase protein synthesis. Insulin stimulates DNA and RNA, thereby increasing the enzymes responsible for protein synthesis. Proof of insulin's effect on protein synthesis has come from many studies. Investigators from Penn State University Medical School showed that insulin stimulated the cellular machinery (ribosomes) involved in the manufacture of protein. In another study, researchers from the University of Texas Health Science Center in Galveston found that, following an insulin infusion, protein synthesis in the muscle cell increased almost 67 percent.

INSULIN INCREASES AMINO ACID TRANSPORT

Although most people are aware that insulin increases glucose transport into muscle cells, most are not aware that insulin also increases amino acid uptake into the muscle. This is important because amino acids are the building blocks of protein. Muscle cell enzymes need a sufficient supply of amino acids to drive protein synthesis. Biolo and his colleagues at the University of Texas Health Science Center in Galveston showed that the infusion of insulin into healthy volunteers increased the rate of transport of key amino acids into the muscle from 20 percent to 50 percent and this increase was associated with enhanced protein synthesis.

INSULIN REDUCES PROTEIN DEGRADATION

Net protein gain is a function of protein synthesis and protein degradation. Net protein gain will occur whenever protein synthesis exceeds protein degradation. Even though there is a strong increase in protein synthesis after exercise, there is also considerable protein degradation. In fact, there is actually a net protein loss. By decreasing protein degradation, we can change this net protein reduction into a net protein gain. Insulin has been shown to suppress protein degradation following exercise, thereby increasing net protein gain.

The takeaway message from these studies is that insulin can increase net protein gain by increasing amino acid transport, increase protein synthesis, and decrease protein degradation, as illustrated in Figure 3.1.

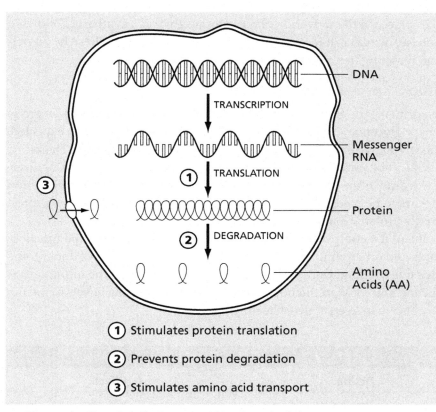

DNA

TRANSCRIPTION

Messenger RNA

① TRANSLATION

③

Protein

② DEGRADATION

Amino Acids (AA)

① Stimulates protein translation

② Prevents protein degradation

③ Stimulates amino acid transport

Figure 3.1. How Insulin Increases Net Protein Gain
Insulin can increase net protein balance by 1) stimulating protein synthesis at the level of mRNA translation, 2) decreasing the degradation of protein, and 3) stimulating the transport of amino acids into the muscle cell.

INSULIN INCREASES GLUCOSE UPTAKE

Insulin's ability to increase glucose uptake is its best-known action. Following exercise, the metabolic machinery is involved in replenishing muscle glycogen. Insulin shuttles glucose into the muscle where it can then be converted into glycogen by muscle cell enzymes. After exercise, the muscle is very receptive to insulin stimulation of glucose uptake.

INSULIN INCREASES MUSCLE GLYCOGEN STORAGE

During resistance exercise, muscle glycogen stores can be significantly reduced. Aside from creatine phosphate (CP), glycogen is the primary fuel for the replenishment of ATP. The conversion of glucose into glycogen takes place via the activation of the enzyme glycogen synthase. Following exercise, insulin can increase the activity of glycogen synthase by 70 percent, resulting in a tremendous increase in glycogen storage.

INSULIN SUPPRESSES CORTISOL RELEASE

The primary trigger for cortisol release during prolonged aerobic exercise is hypoglycemia, or reduced blood glucose levels. This is to be expected, since hypoglycemia is a metabolic stress to the nervous system. Therefore, it is also not surprising that carbohydrate supplementation during exercise would blunt the rise in cortisol, and this cortisol-blunting action appears to be mediated by insulin. Higher insulin concentrations protect muscle protein from the catabolic effects of cortisol.

Insulin's effect on cortisol may also help maintain immune function. Colds and other viral infections are quite common in athletes undergoing intensive training. Cortisol has been shown to suppress the immune system and antibody production. Thus, the cortisol-blunting effects of insulin may also help keep athletes healthy.

TABLE 3.2. Insulin's Anabolic Actions

Action	Effect
Protein synthesis	Increases
Amino acid transport	Increases
Protein degradation	Decreases
Glucose uptake	Increases
Glycogen storage	Increases
Cortisol release	Decreases
Muscle blood flow	Increases

INSULIN INCREASES MUSCLE BLOOD FLOW

Another, less well-known but essential effect of insulin is on muscle blood flow. Insulin infusion has been shown to increase skeletal muscle and limb blood flow by more than 100 percent. Insulin not only increases muscle blood flow, but it targets specific muscles that have been exercised. Increased blood flow results in faster removal of metabolic wastes, such as lactic acid and carbon dioxide, and an increased delivery of nutrients, such as amino acids, glucose, and oxygen, for a more rapid recovery from exercise.

SUMMARY

Hormones are the agents that drive muscle development. They are classified as catabolic and anabolic. Catabolic hormones, including glucagon, epinephrine, norepinephrine, and cortisol, are involved in breaking down nutrients primarily for use as energy. Anabolic hormones—including testosterone, growth hormone, IGF-1, and insulin—are involved in the replenishment of fuel stores and the repair, rebuilding, and growth of muscles.

Contrary to popular belief, insulin is the most powerful anabolic hormone—the most important hormone of all in relation to muscle growth. It is not all good all the time, however. If you are sedentary and have a high-carbohydrate diet, insulin can increase fat stores. But if you are a strength athlete who trains smart and practices the Nutrient Timing System correctly, you will find yourself harnessing the great power of insulin to achieve your goal of gaining muscle mass and strength and keeping your body fat level very low. In Part III, you are going to learn exactly how to employ the Nutrient Timing System to take full advantage of this anabolic controller. Turn now to Part II for a complete discussion of the three NTS phases.

KEY TAKEAWAYS

- Muscle growth and activity are controlled in large part by anabolic and catabolic hormones.

- The primary catabolic hormones are glucagon, epinephrine, norepinephrine, and cortisol.

- The primary anabolic hormones are testosterone, growth hormone, IGF-1, and insulin.

- Following exercise, muscle cells are especially sensitive to the multiple anabolic effects of insulin.

- Insulin increases muscle glucose uptake and glycogen storage.

- Insulin increases net muscle protein by increasing amino acid transport into the muscle cell, by increasing protein synthesis and by reducing protein breakdown.

- Because of its impact on so many muscle anabolic processes, insulin is truly "the anabolic controller."

- The principles of Nutrient Timing can help you maximize the effects of the anabolic hormones while minimizing the effects of catabolic hormones.

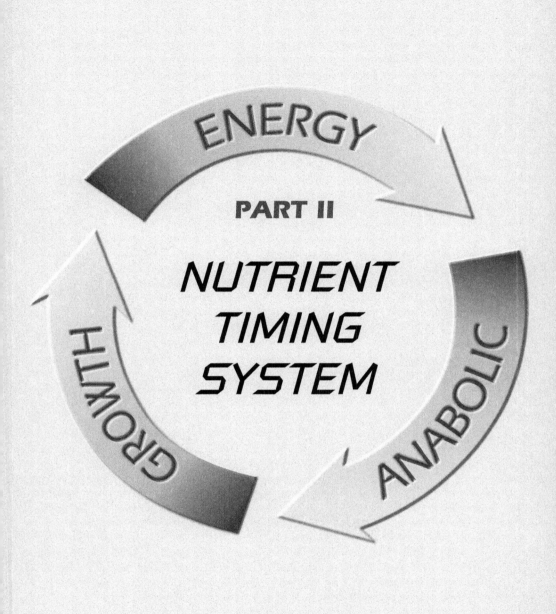

ENERGY

PART II

NUTRIENT TIMING SYSTEM

ANABOLIC

GROWTH

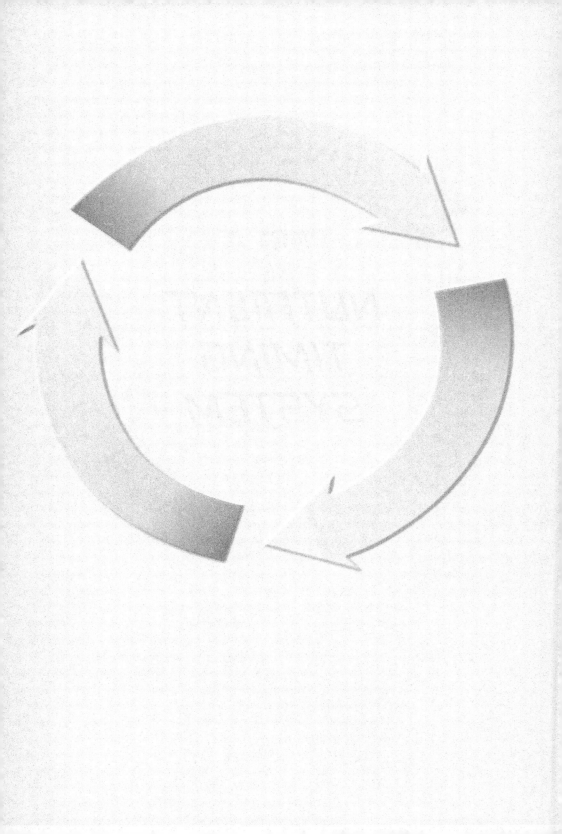

NTS Energy Phase

The Energy Phase of the Nutrient Timing System is the period of your workout. The objective of a resistance workout is to repeatedly require the muscles to generate high levels of force, which requires a high rate of energy release. This chapter explains how the principles of Nutrient Timing will help you produce the energy needed to achieve a stronger workout, how to minimize muscle damage that occurs as a natural consequence of exercise, and, most important, how to set the stage for a faster recovery following your workout.

PHYSIOLOGICAL AND METABOLIC CHANGES DURING EXERCISE

Exercise stresses many systems of the body. At the onset, there is an immediate need to produce greater amounts of energy; as exercise intensity increases, so do the muscles' energy requirements. To accommodate these increased energy needs, the body must initiate multiple physiological and metabolic changes. While these changes are essential for providing an adequate supply of energy to the working muscles, they may also result in transient adverse effects such as muscle damage and immune system suppression. Let's consider some of the more important changes and their consequences.

ATP Replenishment

Muscle fibers need a rapid supply of energy during a resistance workout. This requires the utilization of large numbers of ATP molecules. The breakdown of ATP releases the energy that directly drives muscle contraction. There is, however, only enough ATP stored in the muscle for a few seconds of maximal effort. Therefore, ATP has to be rapidly and continuously replenished during repetitive or sustained muscle contractions.

The primary sources for rapid repletion of ATP during intense exercise are creatine phosphate (CP) and muscle glycogen. Unfortunately, CP stores in the muscle are also quite limited and are depleted with just ten to twelve seconds of maximum-intensity work. If you combine the amount of ATP stored in the muscle and the amount of CP available to replenish ATP, you have only enough energy to drive exercise for twelve to eighteen seconds.

The rapid repletion of ATP and CP involves the anaerobic energy system, or glycolysis. As discussed in Chapter 2, in the anaerobic energy system, muscle glycogen is broken down to generate ATP. Most strength athletes do not realize how much muscle glycogen is used during a training session. One set of ten biceps curls results in a 12 percent loss of muscle glycogen; three sets result in 35 percent depletion, and six sets result in 40 percent depletion.

Hormonal Changes

During resistance exercise there are changes in a number of key hormones. Anabolic hormones such as testosterone, growth hormone, and IGF-1 are elevated for a short period of time and are not believed to play a major role during exercise. There is also a rise in epinephrine and norepinephrine, two catabolic hormones that increase the breakdown of muscle glycogen and fat for energy.

The two most important regulatory hormones during exercise are insulin and cortisol. The opposing actions of these two hormones affect the degree of muscle damage and glycogen depletion during exercise. In the absence of nutritional supplementation, insulin levels decline during exercise while levels of cortisol begin to rise.

Blood Flow

Because of the increased energy and nutrient needs of the muscle, blood flow to active muscles is elevated up to 500 percent. This elevated blood flow results in faster delivery of oxygen and fuel and faster removal of metabolic wastes such as lactic acid and carbon dioxide.

Effect on the Protein Pool

During sustained exercise, a net muscle protein loss occurs. This is mainly because there is an increased use of branched-chain amino acids (BCAAs) for energy. BCAAs are generated by muscle protein breakdown. Because BCAAs serve as precursors for the synthesis of glutamine, muscle glutamine stores decline as well. Glutamine, the most abundant amino acid in muscles, plays an important role in providing fuel for the immune system. During prolonged stressful exercise, glutamine stores can be almost completely depleted, potentially compromising immune system function.

Muscle Damage

Muscle damage is perhaps the most significant physiological effect of a resistance workout. Exercise physiologists measure muscle damage by using a number of key biochemical markers such as 3-methylhistidine, creatine phosphokinase (CPK), and lactate dehydrogenase (LDH). Because 3-methylhistidine is only found in the muscle contractile protein, its presence in the urine indicates that the muscle fibers have been damaged. Like 3-methylhistidine, CPK and LDH are usually found only within the muscle fiber but appear in the blood when muscle fiber membranes are damaged.

There is no single cause of exercise-related muscle damage. The three primary causes are physical, hormonal, and biochemical. Initial damage occurs as a result of physical forces acting on the muscle cell. Eccentric exercise, in which muscle fibers lengthen while contracting, places great stress on the muscle fibers, resulting in an overstretching and tearing of the contractile proteins, which can lead to inflammation. Some of this damage may be beneficial since it stimulates remodeling of muscle cell fibers, which ultimately results in strength and mass gains. William Kraemer of the University of Connecticut coined the term *muscle tissue disruption* to describe this type of damage because the muscle tissue can recover within twenty-four hours and isn't compromised in its ability to adapt to training.

The second cause of muscle damage is hormonal—specifically, the hormone cortisol stimulates muscle protein breakdown.

The third cause of muscle damage is the generation of free radicals (highly reactive molecules that can damage muscle protein). Free radicals may come from the mitochondria, from the capillaries, or even from specific types of cells associated with the immune system. Regardless of their origin, free radicals can damage cell membranes and may indirectly inactivate key enzymes associated with proper functioning of the immune system.

Acute Inflammatory Response

The acute inflammatory response is the body's response to tissue injury, whether it's caused by exercise, an ankle injury resulting from a fall, or even a cut. Within hours of an injury, specific cells called neutrophils migrate to the site of the damage, where they begin to remove tissue debris. This process causes inflammation and swelling, which further damage muscle cell membranes. The acute inflammatory response continues for a considerable period of time after exercise (which is one reason why muscle soreness often isn't felt for twenty-four hours or more).

Immune Response

Resistance exercise triggers a strong immune response. The immune system responds anytime there is cellular damage, whether it is caused by a virus, a wound, or exercise. The immune system's response to the different types of injuries is quite similar. There is an increase in white blood cells, an increase in natural killer (NK) cells, and an increase in T cells, important fighters of infection. However, during strenuous exercise, there is suppression of the immune system as evidenced by a decrease in the number of T cells and NK cells. This suppression has been found to be intensity- and duration-related. The higher the relative exercise intensity and the longer it is performed, the greater the suppression of the immune system. Immune system suppression can last up to seventy-two hours following exercise and may increase your susceptibility to infection.

Fluid Loss

Water, of course, is a vital nutrient that serves many functions. It is the major constituent of blood. Consuming water during exercise helps maintain blood volume, lower body temperature, and reduce stress on the heart. For the endurance athlete, because dehydration represents the number one physiological risk during exercise, the number one nutritional objective is fluid replacement. For an endurance athlete, a loss of 2 percent body water (3.6 pounds for a 180-pound athlete) will compromise performance. In sports such as football, basketball, and soccer, fluid losses exceeding 2 percent of body weight are frequently observed.

Resistance exercise does not produce fluid losses to the degree that extended aerobic exercise does, but dehydration is still a factor. In a study from Old Dominion University, researchers found that dehydration equal to a 1.5 percent loss of body weight adversely affected strength performance.

Most athletes now recognize the benefits of hydration and even carbohydrate replenishment while training. However, it should now be quite
obvious that the metabolic processes occurring during resistance exercise
require more intensive nutrient intervention (see Table 4.1). As you will see
in the next section, even water with carbohydrates (for example, a typical
sports drink) just doesn't meet the complete nutrient needs of working
muscles.

Table 4.1 summarizes the many physiological and metabolic changes
that take place within the muscle and related systems during intense
exercise.

TABLE 4.1. Physiological and Metabolic Changes During Intense Exercise			
Description	**Change**	**Description**	**Change**
ATP levels	Depleted	Protein degradation	Increased
Muscle glycogen levels	Partially depleted	Muscle damage	Increased
Cortisol levels	Increased	Immune system	Suppressed
Insulin levels	Decreased	Acute inflammatory response	Stimulated
Blood flow to muscles	Increased	Fluid loss	Increased

NTS GOALS FOR THE ENERGY PHASE

The four primary goals of the Nutrient Timing System during the
Energy Phase are:

1. Increase nutrient delivery to muscles and spare muscle glycogen
   and protein.

2. Limit immune system suppression.

3. Minimize muscle damage.

4. Set the nutritional stage for a faster recovery following your
   workout.

1. Increase Nutrient Delivery to Muscles and Spare Muscle Glycogen and Protein

Although glycogen depletion has traditionally been the concern of endurance athletes, it is also an important issue for strength athletes. Muscle glycogen levels following multiple sets can be reduced as much as 40 percent. Doubling the intensity of the workout doubles the breakdown.

ATP and creatine phosphate provide most of the energy for muscle contraction, but glycolysis still plays an important role. Between sets, muscle cells use the glycolytic pathway to regenerate ATP. By consuming a carbohydrate or carbohydrate/protein sports drink during your workout, you can preserve muscle glycogen and remain strong throughout your workout.

Haff and colleagues studied the effect of carbohydrate supplementation during resistance exercise. They found that when the carbohydrate supplements were provided, the decline in muscle glycogen was 50 percent less and that subjects could perform more work than subjects receiving flavored water.

The latest research now shows that the addition of protein to a carbohydrate supplement during resistance exercise offers further advantages in terms of preserving muscle protein, increasing protein synthesis, and even extending endurance.

During extended exercise, amino acids—principally the BCAAs: leucine, isoleucine, and valine—may supply up to 15 percent of the muscles' energy needs. The use of some BCAAs for energy can be increased by as much as 500 percent, depending on the intensity and duration of the exercise. The addition of protein to a carbohydrate supplement promotes the metabolism of the ingested protein and lessens the demand for amino acid release from the muscles.

Recent studies coming out of the University of Texas Health Science Center in Galveston suggest that when protein is added to a carbohydrate supplement and provided at the beginning of exercise, there is even an increase in protein synthesis after exercise.

Finally, the addition of protein to a carbohydrate supplement has been shown to extend muscular endurance. Researchers from the University of Texas in Austin found that a carbohydrate/protein drink improved endurance 57 percent compared with water and 24 percent compared with a carbohydrate-electrolyte drink (see Figure 4.1). The improvement in endurance was thought to be due to a sparing of muscle glycogen and possibly to the preferential metabolism of the ingested protein.

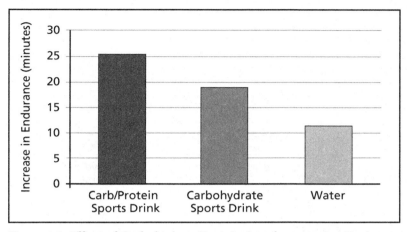

Figure 4.1. Effect of Carbohydrate/Protein Supplementation During Exercise
Following variable intensity exercise, subjects receiving a carbohydrate/protein sports drink had a 24 percent improvement in exercise endurance compared with a carbohydrate sports drink and a 57 percent improvement compared with water. *(Adapted from Ivy et al.)*

2. Limit Immune System Suppression

A second objective of the NTS during the Energy Phase is limiting immune system suppression. During moderate-intensity exercise, immune function is heightened, increasing resistance to infection. However, as discussed, with strenuous exercise, the immune system is suppressed, and the risk of infection is thereby increased.

The immune system is closely linked to the neuroendocrine system, which controls the release of hormones. During strenuous and sustained exercise, this system is activated, causing the release of cortisol. Most of the immunosuppressive responses caused by intense exercise correlate with increases in blood cortisol levels. Cortisol lowers the concentration and activities of many of the important immune cells that fight infection.

Interestingly, blood cortisol levels can be regulated to a significant degree during exercise by controlling glucose availability. Bishop and colleagues showed that when athletes were given a 6 percent carbohydrate solution during exercise, cortisol levels dropped by almost 80 percent compared with subjects receiving water (see Figure 4.2).

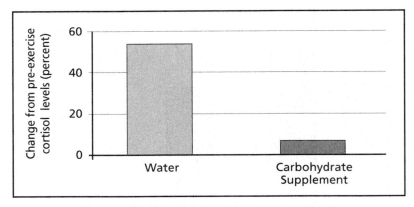

Figure 4.2. Effect on Cortisol Levels of Supplementation During Exercise
When athletes were administered a 6 percent carbohydrate solution during exercise, blood cortisol levels dropped almost 80 percent. *(Adapted from Bishop et al.)*

Because of the high correlation between cortisol and immune system suppression, it is logical that carbohydrate supplementation would limit the suppressive effects of exercise on the immune system. In fact, this has been confirmed, most notably by David Nieman and colleagues at Appalachian State University. These researchers have compared a number of immune system parameters during exercise with and without carbohydrate supplementation. They found that subjects receiving carbohydrate supplementation during intense exercise had lower blood cortisol levels and limited immune suppression—as indicated by a lessened T cell and NK cell reduction—compared with subjects receiving a placebo.

Carbohydrate supplementation provides a dual benefit during exercise, as seen in Figure 4.3. Maintaining blood glucose helps maintain immune function while decreasing cortisol levels.

During resistance exercise, cortisol levels can increase fivefold. Strength athletes who ignore the benefits of nutrient supplementation during their workouts place themselves at a greater risk of experiencing the immune-suppressive effects of cortisol, which include a transient weakening of the body's major mechanisms of fighting infection.

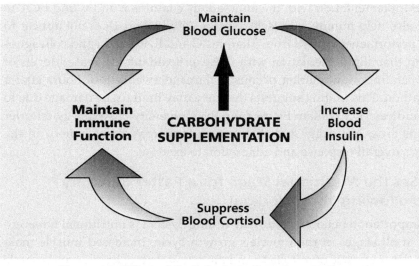

**Figure 4.3. Effect of Carbohydrate Supplementation on
Immune Function**
Carbohydrate supplementation during exercise may help maintain immune function two ways: Carbohydrate supplementation decreases cortisol levels and provides energy to support
the immune system.

It is also important to note, as we will see again in discussing the
Growth Phase (Chapter 6), that strength athletes who severely restrict
their daily carbohydrate intake may be more susceptible to infection.

3. Minimize Muscle Damage

The third important objective of Nutrient Timing during the Energy
Phase is to reduce muscle damage. This damage is beneficial to a degree
because it stimulates the remodeling process, which leads to larger and
stronger muscles. However, the damage to the muscles must be repaired
before the remodeling process can begin. Because there is no single cause
of exercise-related muscle damage, nutritional intervention must address
all the causes.

Carbohydrate supplementation during exercise reduces the rise in
cortisol and decreases specific agents responsible for producing inflammation. Bishop and colleagues from Longborough University in England
showed that carbohydrate supplementation could reduce biochemical
markers of inflammation by almost 50 percent.

Supplementation with the antioxidant vitamins E and C and BCAAs may also help minimize muscle damage. While there does not appear to be a performance benefit from vitamins C and E, Rokitzki and colleagues found that supplementation with these antioxidants decreased levels of CPK, an important marker of muscle damage, twenty-four hours after a marathon. This finding suggests that they may limit tissue damage due to free radicals. Dr. William Evans from the University of Arkansas, a leader in this area, has suggested that antioxidants may be of benefit in the body's overall response and adaptation to exercise.

4. Set the Nutritional Stage for a Faster Recovery Following Your Workout

An important tenet of the Nutrient Timing System is nutritional intervention at all stages in the muscle's growth cycle. Increased muscle mass comes from a cycle of muscle stimulation, muscle breakdown, and muscle rebuilding. Every athlete knows the expression *No pain, no gain*. This is true in the sense that you must train hard enough to cause a degree of muscle tissue disruption. However, training hard without appropriate nutrition intervention results in a more prolonged recovery and ultimately a weaker training response.

Although you cannot entirely prevent muscle damage and depletion of your energy stores during resistance exercise, by applying the principles of the Nutrient Timing System you can minimize these effects, setting the stage for a faster recovery.

As seen above, there is increased muscle protein degradation, in part to help supply muscle energy needs during exercise. Consuming protein during exercise will enable you to utilize the ingested protein and thereby decrease protein degradation and spare muscle protein. The same principle holds true with regard to muscle glycogen. Consuming carbohydrate during resistance exercise results in less depletion of glycogen stores.

The replenishment of muscle glycogen stores is an essential cellular function that is given a metabolic priority by the muscles' anabolic machinery following exercise. The faster this process occurs, the quicker the muscle machinery can be reoriented toward the remodeling of your muscle fibers. The replenishment of your energy stores occurs much faster if you have limited their depletion during your workout by supplementing appropriately.

NTS RECOMMENDATIONS FOR THE ENERGY PHASE

Now that you recognize the importance of nutrient consumption during the Energy Phase, we would like you to redefine when your workout actually begins. For most, it begins with your warm-up stretching or first weightlifting repetition. But there are a number of benefits to be gained if you begin your workout instead while you are driving to the gym. Consumption of a carbohydrate/protein drink ten minutes prior to your workout can raise both blood glucose and insulin levels. At the beginning of your workout, there will be an increase in glucose uptake into the muscles for use as energy, resulting in greater sparing of muscle glycogen and an increase in endurance. A second benefit is that consumption of a carbohydrate/protein drink immediately *before* exercise results in greater protein synthesis *after* exercise. A third potential benefit is that by raising the blood glucose level, you may reduce the rise in cortisol, which begins soon after your workout does.

Nutrient supplementation immediately before exercise and continuing every fifteen to twenty minutes during exercise will not only improve your workout but also lay the groundwork for a faster recovery. Water will help replenish fluid, but a carbohydrate drink or, even better, a carbohydrate/protein drink will deliver additional benefits. If you are to take full advantage of the Nutrient Timing System, the ideal drink to consume before and during exercise should contain the ingredients specified in Table 4.2 and described below.

Carbohydrate

Carbohydrate supplementation during exercise not only helps extend endurance, but also limits suppression of the immune system and reduces muscle tissue damage. The ideal carbohydrates to use are high-glycemic ones such as sucrose, glucose, and maltodextrin. Drinks that contain large quantities of fructose may cause gastrointestinal problems.

Protein

Consuming protein during your workout will limit muscle protein degradation. Protein can also work synergistically with carbohydrate to increase blood insulin levels beyond those produced by carbohydrate alone. Protein has been shown to extend exercise endurance and to increase protein synthesis upon cessation of exercise. The protein of choice

TABLE 4.2. Ideal Nutrient Composition of Supplement for the Energy Phase

NTS OBJECTIVE	Nutrient	Amount (per 12 oz water)
• Increase nutrient delivery to muscles and spare muscle glycogen and protein	High-glycemic carbohydrates such as glucose, sucrose, and maltodextrin	20–26 g
	Whey protein	5–6 g
• Limit immune system suppression	Leucine	1 g
	Vitamin C	30–120 mg
• Minimize muscle damage	Vitamin E	20–60 IU
• Set the nutritional stage for a faster recovery following your workout	Sodium	100–250 mg
	Potassium	60–100 mg
	Magnesium	60–120 mg

is whey because it is rapidly absorbed and contains all the essential amino acids, as well as a high percentage of leucine and glutamine, two amino acids that are used extensively during sustained strenuous exercise. The ratio of carbohydrate to protein should be approximately 3–4 grams of carbohydrate to 1 gram of protein, as this formulation is highly digestible.

Leucine

This amino acid may also be of benefit in a sports drink because it not only stimulates insulin in its own right, but also has a positive effect on protein synthesis.

Electrolytes

Sodium, potassium, and chloride are also necessary in an effective sports drink. The addition of electrolytes not only helps replace what's lost due to sweating but also encourages continued fluid consumption because of the salt, which stimulates thirst.

Vitamins

Although many sports drinks contain varying amounts of different vitamins, we recommend adding vitamins E and C because they reduce free-radical levels, an important cause of muscle damage.

Fluids

You should try to fully replace fluid and electrolyte losses that occur during a strength-training workout. Although strength training does not produce the same level of fluid loss as an endurance workout, fluid losses can still be considerable. Drink at least 12 ounces starting ten minutes before and continuing throughout your workout. For maximum effectiveness, consume several ounces of your Energy Phase beverage every fifteen minutes. In warm weather or when conditions are hot, increase your beverage consumption accordingly.

KEY TAKEAWAYS

- *Strength training depletes muscle glycogen, stimulates the acute inflammatory response, increases protein breakdown, and causes muscle damage.*

- *Carbohydrate supplementation during exercise helps maintain immune system function and blunts the rise of cortisol.*

- *Carbohydrate supplementation combined with protein offers additional endurance benefits and also sets the stage for a faster recovery after your workout.*

- *Consuming a carbohydrate/protein supplement ten minutes before your workout will enable you to have a better workout.*

NTS Anabolic Phase

The Anabolic Phase is the most critical phase of the Nutrient Timing System. Following a workout, the muscle machinery is primarily in a catabolic mode. However, it is primed to switch into an anabolic mode if the right stimuli are provided.

The principles of nutrient optimization and metabolic sensitivity are particularly relevant during the forty-five-minute period postexercise. The switch that turns off the catabolic machinery and turns on the anabolic machinery is insulin. During this forty-five-minute period, muscle cells are acutely sensitive to the anabolic actions of insulin. Just providing the right nutrients will exploit this insulin sensitivity and cause a tremendous surge of anabolic activity.

First, let's consider what happens once we stop exercising. Following exercise, the state of the muscle in many ways is similar to that seen during exercise; however, if recovery measures are not taken, this state can actually worsen. ATP and creatine phosphate (CP) levels are depleted, muscle glycogen levels are reduced, and the rise in cortisol seen during exercise continues in the postexercise period, which means that there is heightened catabolic activity. Other catabolic hormones, such as epinephrine and norepinephrine, remain elevated for thirty to sixty minutes and then return to pre-exercise levels. On the other hand, free radicals generated during exercise are present and will attack muscle cell structure, causing damage for many hours after exercise.

The muscle damage that occurred during exercise has stimulated an acute inflammatory response. Specific cells migrate to the site of muscle damage, increasing inflammation and releasing specific proteins that cause additional damage to muscle membranes. Markers of muscle damage like CPK actually reach a peak twenty-four hours after a work-out—further evidence that membrane damage continues in the post-workout period.

As the damaged muscle cell attempts to repair and rebuild, the increase in protein synthesis that you would expect has been observed. However, the rate of protein degradation exceeds the rate of protein synthesis, resulting in a net muscle protein loss. Furthermore, unless specific nutritional actions are taken, this catabolic state can continue for a considerable period of time.

Some essential amino acids, glutamine, and branched-chain amino acids (BCAAs) are also depleted. This depletion is believed to occur because of the use of amino acids in vital metabolic processes. Because BCAAs are a precursor for glutamine synthesis, their use as an energy source may result in lower glutamine levels.

If the above reasons don't arouse your concern about the state of your muscles postexercise, there is one more. Elevated blood flow postexercise supports the rapid removal of metabolic byproducts and faster nutrient and oxygen delivery. Unfortunately, this is a transitory elevation; blood flow quickly returns to its normal resting level, even though the recovering muscle still requires greater oxygen and nutrient delivery.

Considering this fuel depletion and the biochemically compromised state of the muscles following a workout, it is somewhat surprising to look at what a strength athlete typically consumes during recovery. For many, it is just water. For others, it may be a protein drink. Although each provides a benefit, neither is adequate for complete recovery.

THE METABOLIC COST OF NUTRIENT DELAY

The forty-five minutes immediately following exercise (the Anabolic Phase) is the metabolic window of opportunity. At no other time during the course of your day can nutrition make such a major difference in your overall training program. Although the muscle has residual catabolic activity following exercise, it is primed to shift into an anabolic state in the presence of the right nutrients. If you don't exploit this metabolic receptivity, your muscle cells will remain in a catabolic state and even begin to develop insulin resistance. The metabolic window is only open for a short period of time after exercise. Indeed, within minutes after you stop exercising, it begins to close.

Taking in more nutrients outside the metabolic window will not produce the same results. When insulin resistance develops, usually two to four hours after your workout, even the perfect combination of nutrients will be much less effective.

TIMING AND GLYCOGEN REPLENISHMENT

As early as 1988, in a study published in the *Journal of Physiology*, researchers from the University of Texas at Austin showed that the timing of carbohydrate supplementation postexercise had a significant influence on the rate of muscle glycogen storage. They found that when subjects consumed a carbohydrate supplement immediately after exercise, they stored twice as much muscle glycogen in a two-hour recovery period as when they took the same supplement two hours later. Similar results were obtained by researchers at Vanderbilt University, who found that muscle glucose uptake following exercise was three to four times faster when supplementation was given immediately after exercise rather than three hours later.

TIMING AND PROTEIN SYNTHESIS

Stimulation of protein synthesis is essential for all strength athletes. The ineffectiveness of the bulk protein philosophy (more is better) is illustrated when the relationship between timing and optimal protein synthesis is closely examined.

In order for protein synthesis to occur, amino acids must be transported into the cell, where they can be utilized by the metabolic machinery to repair, rebuild, and remodel muscle protein. Muscle amino acid uptake is controlled in part by the blood amino acid levels. In addition, the level of amino acids in the blood is a critical initiator of protein synthesis. Research studies show that when the amino acid levels of the blood are reduced to below normal, amino acids are released from the muscle and muscle protein synthesis declines. When the blood amino acid levels are increased above normal, muscle amino acid uptake increases as does muscle protein synthesis.

Activation of protein synthesis by amino acids is most responsive immediately following exercise. Biolo and colleagues found that amino acid uptake and muscle protein synthesis were threefold greater in subjects who had engaged in resistance exercise compared with subjects who had not. Likewise, Okamura and colleagues found that in the postexercise recovery period, protein synthesis was almost 25 percent higher and amino acid uptake almost twice as high when a carbohydrate/protein supplement was given immediately after exercise versus two hours after exercise.

The importance of consuming protein during the Anabolic Phase, however, is best illustrated by the results of a study by Levenhagen and colleagues at Vanderbilt University. These researchers looked at the effect of a carbohydrate/protein supplement on protein synthesis following a sixty-minute bout of exercise. Subjects were given the supplement immediately after exercise or three hours later. Protein synthesis was almost three times higher when the supplement was given immediately after, compared with a three-hour waiting period. And the all-important net protein balance (protein synthesis minus protein degradation) increased significantly in the immediate group. In the three-hour group there was actually a net loss of protein. (See Figure 5.1.)

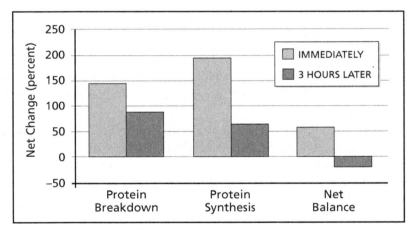

Figure 5.1. Effect of Delay on Net Protein Balance
Subjects were given a carbohydrate/protein supplement either immediately following exercise or three hours after exercise. Receiving supplementation immediately after exercise resulted in an increase in net protein balance, whereas receiving the supplementation three hours after exercise resulted in a net protein loss. *(Adapted from Levenhagen et al.)*

Besides the benefit of increased protein gain, the group receiving the carbohydrate/protein supplement immediately after exercise also had greater fat oxidation—that is, they burned more fat.

TIMING AND INCREASED MUSCLE MASS

Although supplement timing is critical for protein synthesis and net protein balance, it is also important for muscle development. After all, a major goal of most strength athletes is to increase muscle mass.

Using laboratory animals, Suzuki and colleagues were the first to investigate the effects of Nutrient Timing on body composition. They found that when animals were fed right after exercise versus four hours later, muscle weight was higher by 6 percent in the group fed immediately. They also reported that the muscle enzymes responsible for fat oxidation were 70 percent higher and abdominal fat was 24 percent lower in the group immediately fed. The researchers suggested that, compared with nutrient supplementation several hours later, the consumption of nutrients after exercise may contribute to an increase in muscle mass and a decrease in adipose (fat) tissue.

Similar results were seen in a recent human trial by Esmarck and colleagues. In a twelve-week training study published in the *Journal of Physiology*, they reported that when a carbohydrate/protein mixture was given immediately after each exercise session, muscle size increased 8 percent and strength improved 15 percent. When the supplement was given two hours later, there was no muscle hypertrophy (growth) or improvement in strength.

The evidence is overwhelming. Consumption of nutrients during the Anabolic Phase can help you replenish glycogen stores faster, increase protein synthesis and net protein balance, improve muscle mass, and even speed up fat oxidation. But not just any nutrients will do. Although drinking a sports drink is preferable to drinking water, consuming that alone will cost you a great opportunity to improve muscle development. You must consume all of the critical nutrients in the right proportions while the metabolic window is open.

The two conditions for muscle growth are metabolic sensitivity and nutrient optimization. The first condition is satisfied in the postexercise interval because your muscle cells are ready to begin the rebuilding and recovery process. For nutrient optimization, all you have to do now is consume all of the nutrients necessary to drive recovery.

NTS GOALS FOR THE ANABOLIC PHASE

The five goals of the Nutrient Timing System during the Anabolic Phase are:

1. Shift metabolic machinery from a catabolic state to an anabolic state.

2. Speed the elimination of metabolic wastes by increasing muscle blood flow.

3. Replenish muscle glycogen stores.

4. Initiate tissue repair and set the stage for muscle growth.

5. Reduce muscle damage and bolster the immune system.

All of this sounds pretty complicated, but it's not. Once again, the science shows that these goals are readily achievable by following some simple steps.

1. Shift Metabolic Machinery from a Catabolic State to an Anabolic State

In Chapter 3, you learned how important insulin is in regulating anabolic processes. Now, the most effective way to stimulate insulin release is to ingest high-glycemic sugars, right? Not exactly. While ingesting carbohydrate alone will accomplish the goal, it is nowhere near as effective as using a carbohydrate/protein supplement.

Use of a carbohydrate/protein supplement will stimulate insulin and blunt cortisol release. The synergistic effects of carbohydrate and protein were first noted almost forty years ago. In an effort to determine the effect of food on insulin secretion, scientists noted that foods high in protein, when combined with carbohydrates, raised blood insulin levels more than other food combinations. Spiller and colleagues later followed up on this research by comparing the insulin response to carbohydrate drinks and carbohydrate/protein drinks. They showed that the addition of protein to a carbohydrate drink produced a far greater insulin response than a carbohydrate drink alone.

Researchers at the University of Texas at Austin extended these findings by comparing the effects of carbohydrate, protein, and carbohydrate/protein supplements on blood insulin levels after exhaustive exercise. The carbohydrate/protein drink produced the greatest insulin response followed by the carbohydrate drink and then the protein drink. (See Figure 5.2.) In fact, the protein supplement by itself produced one-eighth as much insulin response as the carbohydrate/protein combination. Not only did the carbohydrate/protein produce a greater response, but it was also found that this response could be maintained throughout the recovery period with continued supplementation to drive postworkout anabolic processes.

Stimulating insulin release is the first step in shifting the metabolic machinery to an anabolic state after exercise. Once high levels of insulin are achieved, a number of anabolic reactions are activated in the presence of the right nutrients.

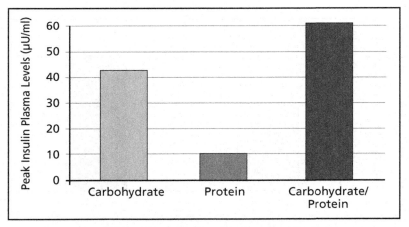

Figure 5.2. Effect of Supplementation Type on Insulin Response
Effect of carbohydrate, protein, and carbohydrate/protein supplementation on blood insulin levels after exhaustive exercise. A carbohydrate/protein supplement produced the greatest insulin response. *(Adapted from Zawadzki et al.)*

2. Speed the Elimination of Metabolic Wastes by Increasing Muscle Blood Flow

Recovering muscle requires fast nutrient and oxygen delivery as well as fast removal of metabolic byproducts such as lactic acid. Removal of lactic acid is particularly important to the recovery of creatine phosphate (CP), the main precursor by which ATP is regenerated during resistance exercise. When lactic acid levels are high, it takes longer for CP to be restored. One of the little known but important effects of insulin is the increase of skeletal muscle blood flow. Laakso and colleagues showed that insulin could increase muscle blood flow approximately twofold (see Figure 5.3).

The mechanism by which insulin increases skeletal muscle blood flow involves nitric oxide synthesis. Nitric oxide (NO) has lately received a lot of attention as a means to induce vasodilation (increased blood flow) in muscle. The precursor for NO is the amino acid arginine. A number of arginine products are currently available from manufacturers who tout their ability to increase NO production. Studies suggest that insulin is also a strong stimulator of the NO pathway. In one study, insulin infusion into the blood was shown to be more effective in increasing NO-dependent muscle blood flow than 30 grams of arginine.

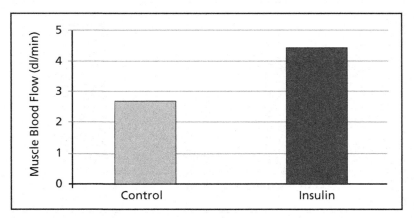

Figure 5.3. Effect of Insulin on Muscle Blood Flow
Following insulin infusion, muscle blood flow almost doubled when compared with muscle blood flow in a control group. *(Adapted from Laasko et al.)*

3. Replenish Muscle Glycogen Stores

Some of the most important studies on exercise recovery have measured the effects of carbohydrates on the replenishment of muscle glycogen stores postexercise. These studies have found that supplementing with carbohydrate immediately after exercise is much more effective than delaying supplementation. It has also been found that supplementing on a regular basis after exercise can maintain a rapid rate of glycogen storage during the early hours of recovery, and that carbohydrates that produced the greatest insulin response also produce the highest rates of glycogen storage. In fact, the rate of muscle glycogen storage postexercise appears to be directly related to the blood insulin response. That is, the higher the insulin response the greater the rate of muscle glycogen synthesis.

Trying to increase the blood insulin level by simply increasing the carbohydrate content of the supplement was initially effective, but only up to a point. When the carbohydrate content of the supplement exceeded 0.5 grams of carbohydrate per pound of body weight per hour, both the blood insulin response and the rate of muscle glycogen synthesis plateaued.

After this plateau effect was discovered, a number of investigators, knowing that by stimulating a greater amount of insulin they would probably also stimulate a stronger surge in anabolic activity, began to investigate whether they could increase the level of insulin by adding one or more additional nutrients to carbohydrates.

In a pivotal study at the University of Texas at Austin, researchers demonstrated that adding protein to a carbohydrate supplement could increase the effectiveness of the carbohydrate to stimulate muscle glycogen synthesis by increasing the blood insulin response. The carbohydrate/protein supplement was found to be almost 38 percent more effective in restoring muscle glycogen than a carbohydrate supplement and almost four times more effective than a protein supplement. Using nuclear magnetic resonance spectroscopy, a sophisticated technique that evaluates the rate of muscle glycogen storage, these researchers also showed that a carbohydrate/protein supplement was significantly more effective than a carbohydrate supplement of equal caloric content. Interestingly, during the first forty-five minutes of recovery, muscle glycogen storage for the carbohydrate/protein supplement was two times faster than the carbohydrate supplement containing the same amount of calories.

In another study comparing the effects of a carbohydrate/protein drink to those of a carbohydrate drink, van Loon and colleagues at Maastricht University in the Netherlands found a near doubling of the insulin response to the former that was consistent with a near doubling of muscle glycogen storage.

The importance of rapidly replenishing muscle glycogen was clearly evidenced in a collaborative study that included researchers from North Texas State University School of Medicine and the University of Texas at Austin. When subjects consumed a carbohydrate/protein drink, endurance performance after four hours of recovery was 55 percent greater than when they consumed a carbohydrate drink (see Figure 5.4). The increase in performance was directly related to greater muscle glycogen synthesis during the recovery period. Researchers in the Allied Health Science Center at Springfield College have also documented faster recovery and better performance in a subsequent workout when comparing carbohydrate/protein and carbohydrate supplements.

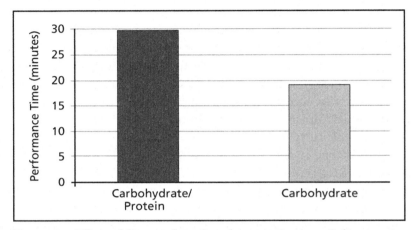

Figure 5.4. Effect of Postworkout Supplementation on a Subsequent Exercise Bout
Following a glycogen-depleting exercise bout, subjects were given either a carbohydrate or a carbohydrate/protein/antioxidant/glutamine beverage. Following a four-hour recovery period, the subjects completed an exercise bout to exhaustion. When the subjects received the carbohydrate/protein/antioxidant/glutamine drink, their performance times in the second workout were 55 percent better than when they received the carbohydrate supplement. *(Adapted from Williams et al.)*

4. Initiate Tissue Repair and Set the Stage for Muscle Growth

Because net protein gain is a sum of both synthesis and breakdown, merely looking at protein synthesis as a measure of net protein gain can be misleading. To increase muscle mass and strength in the postworkout period, the muscle cell must begin to initiate tissue repair and to set the stage for muscle growth.

Researchers at McMaster University in Hamilton, Ontario, reported that supplementing with a carbohydrate/protein supplement, both immediately and one hour after resistance exercise, increased muscle protein synthesis compared with a carbohydrate supplement. They noted higher blood insulin and glucose levels and lower 3-methylhistidine excretion following consumption of the carbohydrate/protein supplement. You may recall that 3-methylhistidine excretion is an indicator of muscle fiber damage.

Additional evidence of the positive effect of a carbohydrate/protein supplement on postexercise protein synthesis comes from Vanderbilt University. Investigators showed that a carbohydrate/protein supplement provided immediately after exercise increased protein synthesis almost sixfold over a carbohydrate supplement. The results for the all-important net protein balance were even more telling. The carbohydrate/protein supplement showed a significant increase in net protein balance compared with the carbohydrate supplement.

Intuitively, you might expect these results since protein synthesis requires amino acids, which obviously are not found in a carbohydrate supplement. A more interesting comparison would be between a carbohydrate/protein supplement and a protein supplement. The answer to this question comes from a recent study from the University of Texas Health Science Center at Galveston. Scientists evaluated the effects of a carbohydrate supplement, an amino acid supplement, and an amino acid/carbohydrate supplement on protein synthesis. The results were dramatic. As shown in Figure 5.5 on page 58, the researchers found that protein synthesis was greatest with the carbohydrate/amino acid supplement and least with the carbohydrate supplement. In fact, the carbohydrate/amino acid supplement was 38 percent more effective than the amino acid supplement and 100 percent more effective than the carbohydrate supplement. This study, more than any other study, should convince you that that the combination of carbohydrate and protein produces a synergistic effect on protein synthesis.

Consumption of a carbohydrate/protein drink postexercise may also replenish glutamine stores faster. Schoore and his colleagues from the University of Maastrich in The Netherlands provided either a carbohydrate/protein supplement or a carbohydrate supplement one and two hours after exercise. Plasma glutamine levels decreased 20 percent in subjects receiving the carbohydrate alone and remained low in recovery (see Figure 5.6 on page 58). In subjects consuming the carbohydrate/protein supplement, postexercise glutamine levels did not decline.

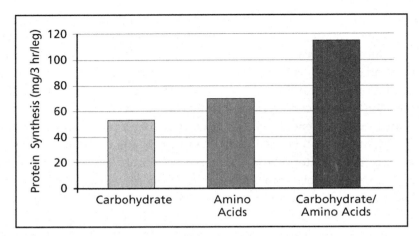

Figure 5.5. Effect of Amino Acids and Carbohydrate Mixture on Protein Synthesis Following Exercise

Following resistance exercise, subjects received either a carbohydrate, amino acid, or carbohydrate/amino acid supplement. The carbohydrate/amino acid mixture increased protein synthesis 38 percent more than the amino acid mixture and 100 percent more than the carbohydrate supplement. *(Adapted from Miller et al.)*

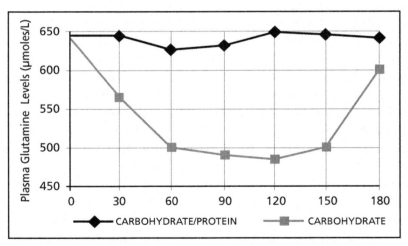

Figure 5.6. Glutamine Levels with Carbohydrate versus Carbohydrate/ Protein Supplementation

Subjects receiving a carbohydrate/protein supplement following exercise were able to maintain plasma glutamine levels, whereas subjects receiving carbohydrate alone had a 20 percent decrease during the first hour following exercise. *(Adpated from Schoore et al.)*

5. Reduce Muscle Damage and Bolster the Immune System

The final goal of Nutrient Timing in the Anabolic Phase is to reduce muscle damage and stimulate the immune system. There is no way to eliminate all the muscle damage resulting from resistance exercise. In fact, to do so would even be undesirable since muscle damage serves as a stimulus for muscle growth. However, excessive muscle damage will restrict glycogen and protein synthesis, cause excessive muscle soreness, and delay recovery. Therefore, to the degree that you can limit muscle damage and reduce muscle soreness, you can come back stronger the next day. Here again, nutrition in the postexercise period plays a role. Using a carbohydrate/protein drink that also contained vitamins E and C and glutamine, researchers found a significant reduction in free-radical formation compared with a plain carbohydrate supplement.

Using this same multi-nutrient beverage composition, Siefert and colleagues at St. Cloud University reported a 37 percent reduction in blood CPK, an important marker of muscle damage, after a prolonged exercise bout (see Figure 5.7).

One of the most exciting examples of how nutrition can reduce muscle inflammatory responses and positively impact the immune system

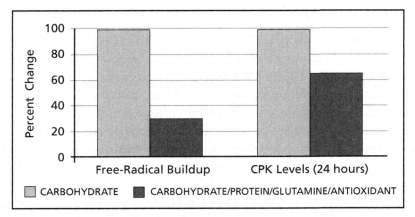

Figure 5.7. Effect of a Carbohydrate/Protein Drink Containing Antioxidants and Glutamine on Parameters of Muscle Damage
Subjects were given either a carbohydrate or a carbohydrate/protein/glutamine/antioxidant supplement immediately after exercise. Free radicals were reduced 69 percent and CPK levels were reduced 36 percent at twenty-four hours postexercise.

comes from a recent collaborative study conducted by researchers from Iowa State, Vanderbilt University, and the United States Marine Corp. The researchers looked at the effect of placebo (no nutrients), a carbohydrate control, and a carbohydrate/protein supplement taken by Marine recruits after exercise over a fifty-four-day period. Individuals receiving the carbohydrate/protein supplement experienced:

- 33 percent fewer total medical visits.

- 28 percent fewer visits due to bacterial/viral infections.

- 37 percent fewer visits due to muscle joint problems.

- 83 percent fewer visits due to heat exhaustion.

The researchers suggested that the effect of postexercise supplementation with a carbohydrate/protein supplement on the immune system may be related to the increased availability of specific amino acids such as glutamine, and concluded that the postexercise carbohydrate/protein supplement "may not only enhance muscle protein deposition but also has significant potential to positively impact health, muscle soreness and tissue hydration."

NTS RECOMMENDATIONS FOR THE ANABOLIC PHASE

One important takeaway from this chapter is this: Don't wait if you intend to take full advantage of the postexercise recovery window. This is clearly evidenced in Figure 5.8, which summarizes the effects of delayed nutrient supplementation on muscle anabolic activities. Almost every important anabolic activity is reduced after three hours.

Another important lesson is that any nutrition taken during this interval is better than just plain water. However, the Nutrient Timing System is about optimizing muscle growth and development. The studies described in this chapter show that you will receive many more benefits if your postexercise meal contains the right combination of nutrients. Here are the nutrients/supplements we recommend during the Anabolic Phase.

Whey Protein

Whey protein offers a number of advantages. It contains all nine essential amino acids. It is extremely digestible. It has a higher concentration of

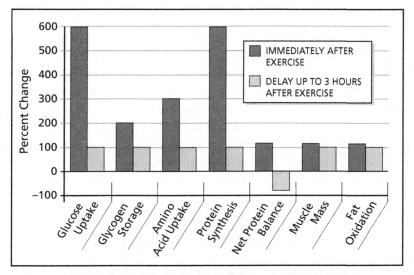

Figure 5.8. Effect of Nutrient Delay on Muscle Anabolic Processes
A delay in nutrient supplementation of up to three hours can dramatically decrease important anabolic activities including glycogen storage and protein balance.

BCAAs than any other protein source. It is fast acting because it empties from the stomach and is absorbed into the bloodstream faster than other proteins. It also contains precursors for the body's natural antioxidants, which may help minimize free-radical formation. Whey protein is readily available and relatively inexpensive.

A disadvantage of whey protein is that it contains lactose. However, lactose-free whey-protein products, which contain lactose amounts of less than 1 percent, are now available.

High-Glycemic Carbohydrates

High-glycemic carbohydrates, which are rapidly absorbed and produce a strong insulin response, are far preferable to complex carbohydrates, which are absorbed far more slowly. Remember, high-glycemic carbohydrates are the catalysts that drive higher anabolic activity postexercise. High-glycemic carbohydrates ideal for postexercise supplementation include sucrose, maltodextrin, and dextrose. Avoid products containing a high percentage of fructose or galactose. These products are weaker stimulators of insulin.

Carbohydrate/Protein Ratio

Studies show conclusively that a carbohydrate/protein combination is superior in stimulating both glycogen replenishment and protein synthesis to either a carbohydrate or protein supplement alone. Carbohydrate provides a strong stimulus for insulin but also provides substrate for replenishment of muscle glycogen stores. The many studies involving carbohydrate/protein supplements that have been cited in this chapter used different ratios of carbohydrate and protein. Based on a review of these studies, we recommend a 3:1 to 4:1 ratio of high-glycemic carbohydrates to protein—in other words, 3 to 4 grams of carbohydrate per gram of

---

Can Nutrient Timing Reduce Frequency of Colds?

A great deal of research has focused on immune status related to exercise. On the one hand, individuals who regularly perform mild to moderate exercise are healthier. Numerous surveys of fitness enthusiasts, runners, and masters athletes show that 60 to 90 percent feel they experience fewer colds than non-exercisers. Data from a number of epidemiological studies support this viewpoint, showing that regular exercise reduces cold symptoms by almost 50 percent.

The reason for this benefit may be related to the stress hormone cortisol. A well-documented effect of cortisol is suppression of the immune system. In individuals who regularly exercise, there is a smaller increase in cortisol levels, which may mean that those who exercise regularly place less stress on their bodies than those who do not exercise at all. Their bodies have adapted to the stress of exercise.

The situation is quite different for individuals who perform heavy exercise on a regular basis. Studies conducted with elite endurance runners have shown that overtraining lowers resistance to upper respiratory infections. Similar results have also been reported for athletes in other sports. The question is whether heavy exercise leads to temporary changes in immunity.

Researchers call this the "open window" theory, which means that after a hard exercise bout the immune system is temporarily compromised. This appeared to be the case in one study when an important barometer of immune function, natural killer (NK) cells, was measured. NK cells are one of the body's important defenses against viral infection.

protein. Table 5.1 on page 64 compares the effects of different beverages on key metabolic activities following a workout. This table, which synthesizes the findings of many different studies, makes a very compelling case for a carbohydrate/protein supplement as the only way to go.

Amino Acids

Amino acids not only serve as a driving force for protein synthesis postexercise, but specific ones such as leucine and glutamine have additional properties that can help in the muscle-recovery process. Leucine, by itself, helps stimulate protein synthesis. Glutamine is also an excellent candidate

NK cells are highly active cells that combat certain types of viruses. During the open window, which ranges from three to seventy-two hours postexercise, there is a decrease in NK activity. Thus, it is logical to assume that risk of infection may be increased following repeated cycles of heavy exercise.

All is not lost, however. Research shows that nutrient supplementation can play an important role in helping the immune system fight infection. A number of studies have shown that carbohydrate ingestion during exercise helps prevent changes in the immune response. One study showed that carbohydrate ingestion significantly lowers blood cortisol and epinephrine levels. And recent studies suggest that a carbohydrate/protein supplement may be even more effective.

In a study described in detail in this chapter, researchers from Iowa State, Vanderbilt University, and the United States Marine Corp found that individuals consuming a carbohydrate/protein supplement postexercise had 28 percent fewer visits to the doctor due to bacterial or viral infections than those consuming a carbohydrate-only supplement.

In addition to reducing cortisol levels, a carbohydrate/protein supplement has also been shown to increase glutamine levels postexercise. Because of the critical role glutamine plays in supporting immune system function, this may be an additional reason why a carbohydrate/protein supplement heightens an individual's response to infection.

The bottom line is that implementing the principles of the Nutrient Timing System can not only help you exercise better and increase muscle mass, but can also help you stay healthier.

for inclusion in a postworkout drink because muscle glutamine stores are depleted following heavy exercise and glutamine has been shown to play an important role in maintaining a healthy immune system.

Antioxidants

Antioxidant vitamins such as E and C should also be included. A hard workout produces free radicals, which not only cause muscle protein damage but also may even have a negative effect on the body's immune system.

TABLE 5.1. Relative Comparison of Different Beverages Used Postexercise (Anabolic Phase)				
Functional Activity	**Water**	**Carbohydrate/ Electrolyte**	**Protein**	**Carbohydrate/ Protein/ Electrolyte/ Antioxidant**
Restore fluids	√	√	√	√
Restore electrolytes		√		√
Replenish glycogen		√		√√
Stimulate protein synthesis		√	√√	√√√
Increase amino acid uptake			√	√√
Prevent protein degradation		√		√√
Blunt cortisol		√		√
Maintain glutamine levels			√	√√
Stimulate insulin		√√	√	√√√
Bolster immune function		√	√	√√
Reduce muscle damage		√	√	√√

ADDITIONAL CONSIDERATIONS FOR THE ANABOLIC PHASE

Although nutrient supplementation can be taken in the form of a meal or beverage, we know full well that after a hard workout most athletes simply are not hungry. However, if they wait until they are hungry, they will miss the critical forty-five-minute window. In our experience, a beverage is easier to consume; therefore, in Table 5.2, we have formulated the ideal beverage. The beverage should contain between 220 and 260 calories. For most athletes, this amount of energy can be consumed in 12 ounces of water. This guideline works well for athletes weighing up to 170 pounds. Athletes who weigh more should increase the amount by 50 percent. Table 5.2 provides the ingredient composition for the ideal supplement to consume during the Anabolic Phase.

TABLE 5.2. Ideal Nutrient Composition of Supplement for the Anabolic Phase		
NTS OBJECTIVE	**Nutrient**	**Amount**
• Shift metabolic machinery from a catabolic state to an anabolic state	Whey protein	13–15 g
	High-glycemic carbohydrates such as glucose, sucrose, and maltodextrin	40–50 g
• Speed the elimination of metabolic wastes by increasing muscle blood flow	Leucine	1–2 g
• Replenish muscle glycogen stores	Glutamine	1–2 g
• Initiate tissue repair and set the stage for muscle growth	Vitamin C	60–120 mg
• Reduce muscle damage and bolster the immune system	Vitamin E	80–400 IU

KEY TAKEAWAYS

- Begin your Anabolic Phase supplementation within forty-five minutes of completing each workout, or risk missing your metabolic window of opportunity.

- A delay of supplementation of more than two hours can significantly reduce protein synthesis and muscle glycogen replenishment.

- The key to optimum recovery is the hormone insulin, which controls many of the cells' postexercise anabolic processes.

- Although muscle cells are extremely sensitive to the effect of insulin immediately after exercise, they rapidly become insulin resistant. So, waiting until the time of insulin resistance to take the correct nutrients reduces their benefit.

- Make sure your Anabolic Phase nutrition has the right formula to blunt catabolic hormones and stimulate anabolic hormones, increase blood flow (for faster nutrient delivery and waste elimination), replenish muscle glycogen stores, initiate tissue repair, and reduce muscular inflammation.

- A carbohydrate/protein supplement in liquid form is very effective in turning on the muscles' anabolic machinery following a workout.

NTS Growth Phase

The third phase of the Nutrient Timing System is the Growth Phase. This is the eighteen- to twenty-hour period during which the majority of gains in muscle mass and strength occur. Life would be easier for strength athletes if the muscles' anabolic machinery operated in a consistent manner for the full interval between workouts. Unfortunately, this is not the case. There are two discrete time segments within the Growth Phase that can be characterized by the intensity of anabolic activity.

The first, the Rapid Segment, is a period of high anabolic activity, which lasts up to four hours if activated during the Anabolic Phase. The second is the Sustained Segment in which muscle growth continues but at a slower rate. This phase is mainly influenced by your diet.

First let's review what happens to muscles following the Anabolic Phase, the forty-five minutes that follow your workout.

When supplementation does not occur, blood insulin levels will remain low and blood cortisol levels will be elevated. Muscle glycogen will remain depleted. Protein degradation and muscle membrane damage will continue. There is continued damage from free radicals and suppresion of the immune system. But the most important change is that without nutrient intervention muscles start to go from a state of high insulin sensitivity to a state of insulin resistance. Once insulin resistance develops, the ability of your muscle cells to maximize anabolic activity, even in the presence of the right nutrients, is severely compromised. When the cellular machinery becomes insulin resistant, which starts about two hours after exercise, it can continue for sixteen hours or longer.

Now let's assume you recognize the importance of postexercise nutrition and have consumed a carbohydrate/protein drink containing glutamine, leucine, and antioxidants immediately after your workout. So you have done everything right. You have increased the blood insulin level, reduced the blood cortisol level, and turned on the anabolic switch. Now you can relax while the cellular machinery of your muscles replenishes the muscle glycogen stores, repairs damaged tissue, and increase muscle protein. Right?

Unfortunately, this is not what happens. Again, to use the car-engine analogy, in the Anabolic Phase you have turned on the cellular ignition and placed the transmission in forward, but if you don't provide sufficient fuel, your car will soon run out of gas. In this case, running out of gas means running out of enough carbohydrate and protein (amino acids) to maintain an elevated blood insulin level, and stimulate muscle glycogen and protein synthesis. Only by keeping insulin levels elevated can high rates of glycogen storage and protein synthesis be maintained during the Rapid Segment.

RAPID SEGMENT OF THE GROWTH PHASE

An important aspect of Nutrient Timing is that, although the muscle growth cycle occurs in separate phases, in reality supplementation in each phase influences the subsequent phase. Turning on the anabolic switch during the Anabolic Phase is the essential first step, but without continuing the right type of nutrient consumption, this anabolic surge will not be maintained.

The two NTS objectives for the Rapid Segment of the Growth Phase are:

1. Maintain increased insulin sensitivity.

2. Maintain the anabolic state.

1. Maintain Increased Insulin Sensitivity

Researchers at the University of Texas at Austin showed that the ability of the muscle cell to replenish glycogen stores is 50 percent less two hours after exercise than it is immediately after exercise. Levenhagen and colleagues at Vanderbilt University have reported similar results for protein synthesis. When a carbohydrate/protein supplement was given immediately after exercise, muscle protein synthesis was elevated 300 percent, but when the supplement was delayed by three hours, the elevation in synthesis was only 12 percent. These results indicate that the muscle is more insulin sensitive early in the recovery period, and that as time passes, it becomes insulin resistant.

Once the muscle becomes insulin resistant, as we have seen, consuming the right nutrients will not produce the desired effect. In other words, the anabolic processes necessary to rebuild and help the muscles grow will not operate at their optimal rate. This means that additional carbohydrates must be consumed with protein and other essential nutrients. However, this becomes a delicate nutritional balance. You want to consume only enough carbohydrates to make sure that the insulin pump is primed and muscle sensitivity to insulin is not lost.

A review of the literature suggests that in the Anabolic Phase, supplements should be composed of a 3:1 to 4:1 ratio of carbohydrate to protein (3 to 4 grams of carbohydrate per gram of protein) to fully convert the muscle from a catabolic state to an anabolic state. During the Rapid Segment of the Growth Phase, you can capitalize on the insulin response that was initiated during the Anabolic Phase. The question is, what is the ideal quantity of carbohydrate to be added to protein?

The muscles in the typical strength athlete have between 100 grams and 120 grams of glycogen per kilogram of muscle. During a strenuous high-intensity workout, about 40 percent of this stored glycogen will be depleted. If you consume sufficient carbohydrate and protein during the Anabolic Phase, as much as 65 to 75 percent of your glycogen stores are replenished within two hours of completing your workout, with no additional supplementation.

Once this level of glycogen storage is attained, a lower consumption of carbohydrate in conjunction with protein will provide sufficient stimulus to keep blood insulin levels elevated. This will maintain the muscle cells' sensitivity to the anabolic effects of insulin and assure complete recovery of muscle glycogen.

During the Energy and Anabolic Phases, it is almost mandatory that insulin be strongly stimulated to drive protein synthesis and muscle recovery. Figure 6.1(a) on page 70 illustrates the twenty-four-hour cycle of insulin sensitivity in the muscle in the absence of any supplementation

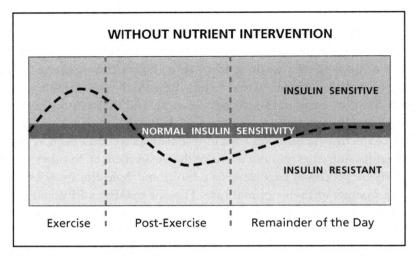

Figure 6.1(a). The Effect of Exercise and Recovery on the Muscle Response to Insulin (without Supplementation)

In the absence of supplementation, the muscles' sensitivity to insulin decreases rapidly. During the postexercise period, muscles become insulin resistant and can remain so for up to sixteen hours if nutrient intake is withheld.

during or after exercise. As you can see, muscles are extremely sensitive to insulin during exercise. This sensitivity decreases without any nutrient intervention and muscles actually become insulin resistant two hours after exercise. This insulin-resistant state can last up to sixteen hours after exercise if nutrient intake is withheld.

Figure 6.1(b) illustrates the goal of nutrient intervention. Consumption of a carbohydrate/protein sports drink during exercise and a carbohydrate/protein recovery drink postexercise prevents the development of insulin resistance, allowing the muscle cells to maintain a high level of anabolic activity. To the degree that you can extend the muscles' insulin sensitivity for up to three to four hours after the Anabolic Phase, you will be rewarded with greater gains in lean muscle mass and strength. It is important to remember that the goal is not to keep blood insulin levels high for the full twenty-four-hour growth cycle. This would not be beneficial. But if you can maintain elevated blood insulin and muscle insulin sensitivity during the Rapid Segment, the benefits to your muscle-development program will be substantial.

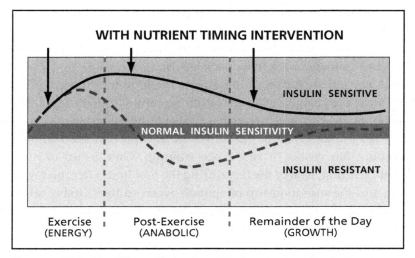

WITH NUTRIENT TIMING INTERVENTION

INSULIN SENSITIVE

NORMAL INSULIN SENSITIVITY

INSULIN RESISTANT

Exercise | Post-Exercise | Remainder of the Day
(ENERGY) | (ANABOLIC) | (GROWTH)

Figure 6.1(b). The Effect of Nutrient Timing on the Muscle Response to Insulin

When nutrient supplementation is supplied during the Energy Phase, Anabolic Phase, and Rapid Segment of the Growth Phase, muscle cells are insulin sensitive for an extended period of time. This extended insulin sensitivity in the presence of nutrient intervention enables the muscle cells to maintain a high level of anabolic activity.

2. Maintain the Anabolic State

The second objective is to maintain the anabolic state for up to four hours after exercise. Among the first to demonstrate that a high level of anabolic activity could be maintained with supplementation after exercise were Blom and colleagues. Their study found that providing a high-carbohydrate supplement immediately after exercise and continuing supplementation at two hours and again at four hours after exercise maintained a high blood insulin level and rapid rate of muscle glycogen synthesis for up to six hours.

A similar pattern was seen with regard to protein synthesis. Rasmussen and colleagues studied the effects of consuming a carbohydrate/protein drink at one hour and again at three hours after a bout of resistance exercise. When the carbohydrate/protein drink was consumed at one hour, there was a sharp rise in insulin, which returned to resting values within one hour. The researchers also found that protein synthesis only increased during the time when insulin was elevated. Thus, the stimulation and decline of protein synthesis paralleled blood levels of insulin. When a second serving of the carbohydrate supplement was given at three hours postexercise, blood insulin rose once again and protein synthesis was stimulated back to its peak levels.

One of the first studies to investigate the long-term effects of maintaining an active anabolic state after exercise comes from the laboratory of Masashigi Suzuki at the University of Wasida in Japan. Suzuki and colleagues fed a high-glycemic carbohydrate and protein meal to animals undergoing ten weeks of resistance training. One group of animals received their first meal of the day during the first hour after their exercise session, and the second group of animals received their first meal of the day during the fourth hour after their exercise session. After the ten weeks of training, there was no difference in weight gain between the two groups of animals; however, muscle mass was 6 percent higher and body fat 25 percent lower in the group fed immediately after exercise. Interestingly, the animals fed immediately after exercise had a higher resting metabolic rate, possibly due to their greater muscle mass.

Leucine may also be helpful in maintaining high anabolic activity during this time. A study conducted by Anthony and colleagues at the University of Illinois found that leucine stimulates muscle protein synthesis following exercise. The effect of leucine on protein synthesis appears to be independent of its effects on insulin. However, when insulin was stimulated by carbohydrate in combination with leucine, there was a further increase in protein synthesis. The authors suggested that leucine in combination with carbohydrate would be useful in helping muscles recover faster.

SUSTAINED SEGMENT OF THE GROWTH PHASE

This segment begins approximately five hours after exercise and continues until your next workout. The time you are sleeping is included in this segment. Your total diet is critically important during this phase. The two NTS objectives for the Sustained Segment of the Growth Phase are:

1. Maintain positive nitrogen balance and stimulate protein synthesis.

2. Promote protein turnover and muscle development.

1. Maintain Positive Nitrogen Balance and Stimulate Protein Synthesis

An essential condition of muscle growth is the maintenance of a positive nitrogen balance. This means that your body is excreting less protein than you are consuming. How much protein does one need to consume in order to maintain a positive protein balance? This is a controversial question. Some nutritionists maintain that the average diet contains more than enough protein for the serious strength athlete. According to the recommended daily allowance (RDA), protein intake should be 0.8 grams per kilogram (2.2 pounds) of body weight per day. The problem is that the nutritionists who developed this recommendation were using sedentary adults as their models. Furthermore, they were not suggesting that this level of protein intake maintains a positive nitrogen balance (positive protein retention), but rather that it maintains a zero nitrogen balance. That is, the amount of protein consumed would prevent a net protein loss, but would not necessarily allow for protein gain.

How much protein should be consumed daily? Obviously, the goal of the strength athlete is not to be in zero nitrogen balance, but to be in positive nitrogen balance. In this regard, Tarnopolsky and colleagues have presented data that indicate a high protein intake will increase nitrogen balance in strength athletes during intense training. Interestingly, a review of the available data indicates that 20 percent of the protein consumed in excess of the maintenance amount is retained. In other words, when more protein is ingested, lean body mass is increased. Moreover, Oddoye and Margen found that a positive nitrogen balance could be maintained for up to fifty days on a diet that was three times the RDA for protein.

So how much protein do we recommend? Fern and colleagues found a greater gain in muscle mass over four weeks of training in bodybuilders who consumed 3.3 grams versus 1.3 grams of protein per kilogram of body weight per day. This suggests that large amounts of dietary protein in combination with strength training will stimulate significant muscle growth. It was also noted that when the bodybuilders consumed the higher protein concentration, a significant amount was oxidized and not retained. This suggests that protein intake exceeded that which could be used for protein synthesis.

In a study by Tarnopolsky and colleagues, an increase in whole-body protein synthesis was observed when strength athletes increased their protein consumption from 0.9 to 1.4 grams per kilogram (g/kg) of body weight per day. However, there was no additional increase in protein synthesis when protein consumption was increased to 2.4 g/kg of body weight per day. Additionally, Lemon and colleagues found that approximately 1.5 g/kg of body weight per day were required to maintain zero nitrogen balance in strength athletes undergoing intense training. Having a positive nitrogen balance required approximately 1.8 g/kg of body weight.

Recently, Forslund and colleagues compared the twenty-four-hour macronutrient metabolism of subjects who had exercised and were on either a high-protein diet (2.5 g/kg of body weight per day) or a normal protein diet (1 g/kg of body weight per day). They found the subjects on the high-protein diet had a positive protein balance and negative fat balance, whereas the subjects on the normal protein diet had zero protein balance and a slight increase in fat balance. In other words, the subjects on the high-protein diet burned more fat.

Table 6.1 summarizes results from multiple studies evaluating the effects of high protein intakes. Based on these studies, we concluded that the strength athlete will receive significant benefits from consuming between 2.0 and 2.75 grams of protein per kilogram of body weight (0.9–1.25 gram of protein per pound of body weight) per day when training intensely. This should be a sufficient amount of protein to maintain a positive nitrogen balance, stimulate muscle growth, and increase reliance on body fat as a fuel source. To make it easy for you to determine your daily protein intake use, Table 6.2 provides the daily protein requirements at protein levels ranging from 0.91–1.25 grams per pound of body weight per day for different body weights.

TABLE 6.1. Studies Evaluating High Protein Intakes

Study	Protein Level(s)	Findings
Fern	3.3 g/kg; 1.3 g/kg	3.3 g/kg protein level produced greater gain in muscle mass
Tarnopolsky et al.	0.9 g/kg; 1.4 g/kg; 2.4 g/kg	Increase in protein synthesis in 1.4 g/kg versus 0.9 g/kg. No additional increase with 2.4 g/kg
Lemon et al.	1.8 g/kg	Required for positive nitrogen balance
Forslund et al.	1.0 g/kg; 2.5 g/kg	2.5 g/kg produced positive nitrogen balance and negative fat balance

TABLE 6.2. Grams of Protein Required According to Body Weight in Pounds

Weight (in pounds)	Daily Protein Level (grams per pound)			
	0.91	1.02	1.14	1.25
125	114	128	143	156
150	137	153	171	188
175	159	179	200	219
200	182	204	228	250
225	205	230	257	281
250	228	255	285	313

2. Promote Protein Turnover and Muscle Development

During the Sustained Segment of the Growth Phase, it is important to continue to promote protein turnover and muscle development. Protein turnover is an essential process in helping build stronger muscles. By definition, protein turnover involves both the processes that break down protein and the processes that build new protein. The reason that protein turnover is an important NTS objective is that when protein turnover is increased, you are rebuilding proteins damaged by training. The result is stronger muscles containing more muscle fibers.

Although protein synthesis will be slower during this segment than during the Rapid Segment, there is still a substantial amount of protein accretion (an increase in protein concentration within a muscle) that can occur during the Sustained Segment of the Growth Phase. According to Fielding and Parkington, protein synthesis may continue after exercise for up to forty-eight hours. However, as we have seen, net protein balance remains negative unless the appropriate foods or amino acid supplements are consumed.

During the Sustained Segment, it is important to maintain elevated blood levels of amino acids, as shown in Figure 6.2 on page 76. This can be done by eating a meal high in protein and snacking between meals with a protein supplement. Researchers have found a positive relationship between the concentration of amino acids in the blood and the rate of protein synthesis. Their results show that increasing protein consumption will increase amino acid levels in the blood and lead to increased protein synthesis.

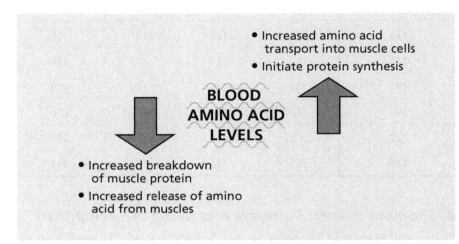

Figure 6.2. Effect of Blood Amino Acid Level on Protein Synthesis and Breakdown
An increase in blood amino acids stimulates amino acid transport into the muscle and increases protein synthesis. When blood amino acid levels are low, there is an increased breakdown of muscle protein and a decrease in overall protein synthesis.

Snacking between meals may be advantageous for several reasons. Results from the University of Texas Health Science Center in Galveston showed that increasing blood amino acid levels improved protein synthesis, but only up to a certain point. After that, the protein-synthesis response failed to increase proportionately. Thus, consuming your protein in one large meal may be much less effective in stimulating muscle protein synthesis than consuming a normal meal and snacking between meals with a high-protein supplement.

In order to maintain a rapid protein turnover rate and rapid muscle growth, it is also important to have a positive caloric balance; in other words, to consume more calories than you expend. There exists substantial evidence indicating that strength athletes can increase muscle mass and strength by simply increasing their caloric consumption. Moreover, there is substantial evidence indicating that a negative caloric balance (consuming fewer calories than are expended) will adversely affect nitrogen retention.

As early as 1907, Chittenden reported that athletes gained strength and maintained mass on relatively low-protein diets as long as sufficient calories were consumed. In addition, Gater and colleagues demonstrated that a positive caloric balance as compared to an equal caloric balance produced the greater gains in muscle mass in subjects undergoing resistance training. Therefore, to maximize your gains in muscle mass, construct your diet so that you consume more calories than you expend.

NTS RECOMMENDATIONS FOR THE GROWTH PHASE

A fundamental principle of the Nutrient Timing System is metabolic sensitivity. By now it should be apparent that the metabolic action of a particular nutrient is highly dependent on when it is consumed. The concept of metabolic sensitivity is illustrated clearly in the nutrient recommendations for this phase.

A carbohydrate/protein supplement is necessary to maintain the anabolic state and heightened level of insulin sensitivity in the four-hour period after your workout. However, once the insulin pump has been primed, less carbohydrate is needed to maintain elevated insulin levels. Whereas a carbohydrate/protein mixture containing more carbohydrate relative to protein (such as 3 to 4 grams of carbohydrate to 1 gram of protein) is ideal to turn on the anabolic machinery, supplementation during the Rapid Segment can rely on a much lower carbohydrate to protein ratio. In fact, 1 gram of carbohydrate to 5–8 grams of protein is appropriate.

Carbohydrate is still needed in amounts sufficient to keep the insulin pump operating at its optimum level. On the other hand, if too much carbohydrate is consumed, it can be converted into fat. Keeping the insulin level elevated for a sustained four-hour period prevents development of insulin resistance, which, as we have seen, will slow or turn off those metabolic processes that are critical for building muscle mass and strength.

It is also recommended that during the Rapid Segment you consume leucine and glutamine because of their anabolic action on protein synthesis and immune system parameters. Table 6.3 on page 78 describes the ideal nutrient composition for a supplement to be used during the Rapid Segment. This nutrient composition will help maintain the high anabolic activity initiated during the Anabolic Phase.

TABLE 6.3. Ideal Nutrient Composition of Supplement for the Growth Phase

GROWTH PHASE	NTS Objective	Nutrient	Amount
Rapid Segment The first 4 hours after a workout	• Maintain increased insulin sensitivity	Whey protein	14 g
	• Maintain the anabolic state	Casein	2 g
Sustained Segment The next 16–18 hours after a workout	• Maintain positive nitrogen balance and stimulate protein synthesis	Leucine	3 g
		Glutamine	1 g
	• Promote protein turnover and muscle development	High-glycemic carbohydrates	2–4 g

During the Sustained Segment of the Growth Phase, insulin levels decline, but it is possible to sustain protein synthesis, although at a slower rate than during the Rapid Segment. This can be accomplished with a proper diet and a carbohydrate/protein snack between meals.

Because your diet represents the bulk of your caloric intake, it has the most influence on protein synthesis and muscle growth during the Sustained Segment. Chapters 7 and 8 detail the NTS daily nutrition plan and help you construct an appropriate plan to meet your goals.

The supplement recommended for the Rapid Segment of the Growth Phase is a high-protein snack that can be used between meals and at bedtime during the Sustained Segment. Such a protein snack or supplement enables you to stimulate protein synthesis by raising the amino acid levels in your blood between meals. As we have shown, elevated amino acid levels stimulate protein synthesis and also slow protein degradation, thereby increasing your net protein balance.

Most important, the high-protein snack does not stimulate insulin. Whereas insulin is essential at specific times, continued elevation of insulin along with high-carbohydrate consumption is not desirable. This insulin elevation can lead to increased fat deposition, elevated blood cholesterol levels, and metabolic disorders.

Protein Type

The objective during both segments of the Growth Phase is to maintain protein synthesis over an extended period of time. Selection of the right type of protein can help you achieve this goal. When comparing the proteins whey and casein, Boirie and colleagues found that protein synthesis increased 68 percent with a whey supplement and 32 percent with a casein supplement. However, the anabolic response of the casein was longer lasting. Because whey is fast acting and the effects of casein are more sustained, we recommend taking a supplement snack composed of both whey and casein during the Growth Phase.

Caloric Balance

Your diet should be in positive caloric balance for muscle repair and growth to be optimized. How large a positive caloric balance will depend on your goals. If you are just trying to gain strength without trying to add much weight, your caloric intake should only exceed your caloric expenditure by 50–100 calories per day. If you are trying to increase mass, you may want your caloric intake to exceed your caloric expenditure by several hundred calories per day. However, if you are a bodybuilder in preparation for competition, you will want to have a negative caloric balance for several weeks leading up to the competition in order to reduce body fat. During this time, you should reduce your carbohydrate intake and increase your protein intake. Table 6.4 summarizes general caloric and nutrient recommendations depending on your specific training goals. However, these are general guidelines. If you find you are not getting the results you want, don't assume that your genes are working against you. If your goal is to gain muscle mass and you are consuming an extra 100–200 calories per day and are not seeing positive results, simply increase your daily caloric intake by another 100–200 calories.

TABLE 6.4. Daily Caloric Consumption and Macronutrient Content Based on Exercise Goals				
Goal	Daily Caloric Balance	Protein	Carbohydrate	Fat
Gain strength	plus 50–100 calories	21–24%	43–46%	33%
Gain lean mass	plus 100–200 calories	21–24%	43–46%	33%
Decrease fat mass	minus 100–200 calories	26%	41%	33%

KEY TAKEAWAYS

- The Growth Phase is the eighteen- to twenty-hour period during which the majority of gains in muscle mass and strength occur.

- The Growth Phase can be subdivided into the Rapid Segment and Sustained Segment.

- The Rapid Segment is a period of high anabolic activity, which can last up to four hours.

- Optimal anabolic activity during the Rapid Segment requires maintaining the high activity initiated during the Anabolic Phase by consuming a carbohydrate/protein supplement approximately two hours after exercise.

- The Sustained Segment is a period of sustained but slow protein synthesis and muscle growth, which extends from the Rapid Segment until the next workout.

- The protein synthesis during the Sustained Segment is strongly influenced by dietary composition and caloric content.

- It is important to maintain a positive nitrogen balance during the Sustained Segment, which can be accomplished with a high-protein diet and high-protein/low-carbohydrate snacks or supplements.

- The strength athlete should consume between 0.91 and 1.2 grams of protein per pound of body weight per day for optimal muscle growth and development.

- A high-protein diet will stimulate a positive protein and carbohydrate balance while causing a negative fat balance.

- A positive caloric balance will also help stimulate protein accretion.

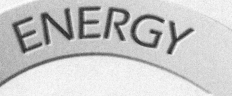

PART III

INCORPORATING NUTRIENT TIMING INTO YOUR TRAINING

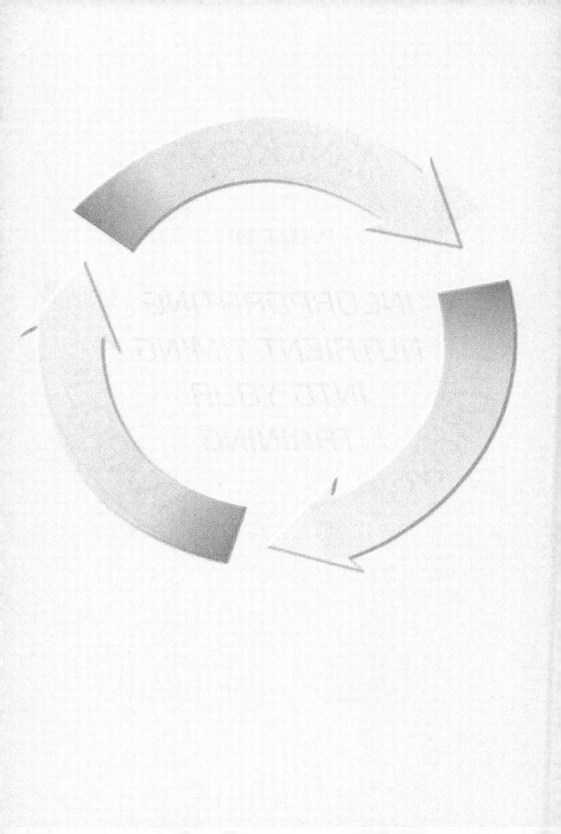

Making Nutrient Timing Work for You

Sports nutrition is skewed toward two ends of the information spectrum. At one end are the nutritionists and "nutritional experts" who advocate a 1960s approach to sports nutrition. Their advice consists mainly of paying attention to the food pyramid, eating lots of leafy vegetables, and trying to control fat intake. According to this approach, you should get all the nutrients you need by following a healthy diet. At the other end of the spectrum are the sports nutrition companies who are often the purveyors of hype. These are the manufacturers who claim their products will "double your lean body mass in a week" while extolling the virtues of their magic herbs and supplements. For them, product claims tend to come out of a thesaurus rather than from a research laboratory. They are the advocates of "more is better." If an ingredient has a benefit, then more of it will give you a greater benefit. Ironically, both of these groups take a similar view of current nutrition research.

For many nutrition traditionalists, good scientific research ended around 1980. They generally fail to incorporate in their programs some of the landmark studies showing how nutrition could have improved the sports performances of the last two decades.

For the purveyors of hype, good scientific research is remote. Their product claims are usually not substantiated by studies, and when they are, the studies may not be relevant to the modern-day athlete's realities.

This information abyss presents a true challenge for the serious strength athlete as he or she tries to navigate through hype and outdated thinking. And of course, most serious athletes are not usually trained in exercise physiology.

We have cited many studies showing the significant and dramatic gains in muscle strength and development that you can achieve by applying a few basic nutrition principles. The science supporting Nutrient Timing is growing; our extensive bibliography at the end of this book is evidence of this growth.

As scientists who are committed to finding safe ways to help improve athletic performance, we find that the most exciting aspect of Nutrient Timing is its power as a tool to help strength athletes achieve their full athletic potential. Figure 7.1 clearly shows the negative impact of nutrient procrastination on most of the muscle cells' key anabolic activities. It also illustrates the positive impact of timely nutrient consumption. Among its other effects, a carbohydrate/protein supplement taken immediately after exercise (versus waiting up to three hours) can result in a 600 percent improvement in protein synthesis and a 100 percent improvement in muscle glycogen replenishment. Following the principles of Nutrient Timing will provide you with the kind of results that will be as powerful as, if not more powerful than, any other sports nutrition program or product.

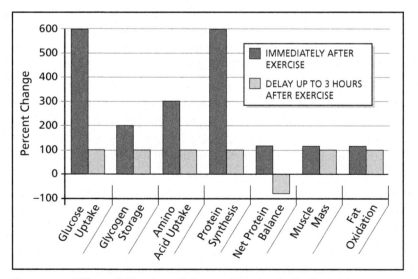

Figure 7.1. Effect of Nutrient Delay on Key Anabolic Activities

However, no matter how strong the science, it must be practical. In other words, Nutrient Timing has to work in the training regimens of strength athletes at all levels and every day. Many pages of this book have

Liquid Nutrition versus Food— Which Provides a Better Recovery?

John M. Berardi, C.S.C.S.

While I believe that complete, unbleached, untreated, and unprocessed whole food should form the basis of a sound nutritional regimen, good nutritional plans for workouts and postexercise recovery are exceptions. Liquid supplemental nutrition may be far superior to whole food for the reasons discussed below.

Liquid Meals Are Palatable and Digestible

Immediately after intense exercise, most people find eating solid food difficult. This is understandable. The stress of exercise creates a situation in which the hunger centers are nearly shut down. However, it's absolutely critical that you eat at this time if you want to remodel the muscle, enlarge the muscle, and recover from the exercise. Fortunately, liquid supplemental formulas are palatable, easy to consume, and can be quite nutrient dense, providing all the nutrition you need at this vital time. In addition, since these formulas are structurally simple, the gastrointestinal tract has no difficulty processing them. Your stomach will thank you.

Liquid Meals Have a Fast Absorption Profile; Whole Food Is Just Too Slow

Liquid supplemental formulas based on the NTS containing fast-digesting protein (whey) and high-glycemic carbohydrates (dextrose and maltodextrin) are absorbed more quickly than whole food. A liquid postexercise formula may be fully absorbed within thirty to sixty minutes, providing your muscles with the essential nutrients during the critical forty-five-minute metabolic window, whereas a solid food meal may take two to three hours to fully affect the muscle.

Liquid Meals Take Advantage of the "Window of Opportunity"; Whole Foods May Miss It

The sooner carbohydrate/protein supplementation gets to the muscles, the better your chances are for muscle building and recovery. The latest research shows that athletes receiving nutrients immediately after exercise recover faster and better than those receiving nutrients two hours later.

Liquid Meals Are Better for Nutrient Targeting

During the postexercise period, an abundance of water and specific nutrients maximize your recovery. These nutrients include high-glycemic carbohydrates, protein (in a specific ratio), and certain amino acids. It's also best to avoid fat during this time. The only way to ensure that these nutrients are present in the right amounts is to formulate a specific liquid blend or buy a commercially available one that meets these criteria. Whole foods may miss the mark, providing too much or not enough of a given nutrient.

---

been devoted to discussing the science underlying the three phases of Nutrient Timing. In this chapter, we fulfill the promise we made in the Introduction. Nutrient Timing is a practical and easy program to implement.

The nutrition foundation for Nutrient Timing is a healthy diet. We offer a number of dietary suggestions and, most important, we have created a template so you can design your own diet based on your own tastes, habits, and lifestyle. To this nutrition foundation, we have added nutrient intervention at three critical times in the muscles' growth cycle: the Energy Phase, the Anabolic Phase, and the Rapid Segment of the Growth Phase. This additional supplementation is usually in the form of a beverage; however, with the exception of the Energy Phase in which hydration is so important, you can create your Anabolic and Growth Phase supplements with the right combination of solid foods. As discussed, there are a number of advantages in taking your nutritional supplementation as a beverage during the four-hour time span that begins just prior to your workout and ends two to three hours after your workout.

The macronutrient requirements for strength athletes looking to get the most out of Nutrient Timing are as follows:

- 19 to 26 percent protein

- 41 to 48 percent carbohydrate

- 33 percent fat

For strength athletes, protein consumption of 0.9–1.2 grams of protein per pound of body weight is ideal. This diet will give you the extra protein you need, which, as we have seen, can help enhance muscle development as well as the necessary energy from carbohydrate and fat to maintain a healthy immune system and minimize the development of overtraining syndrome. (There's more about overtraining in the inset "Overtraining and Nutrition" on page 131 in Chapter 10.)

Table 7.1 shows the nutrient composition at different levels of protein intake for a male weighing 200 pounds and a female weighing 130 pounds.

TABLE 7.1. Daily Nutrient Compositions at Four Levels of Protein Intake

MALE • Weight: 200 pounds • Target Daily Caloric Intake: 3,800

Protein Level (g/lb)	Protein Composition			Carbohydrate Composition			Fat Composition		
	Calories	Grams	Percent	Calories	Grams	Percent	Calories	Grams	Percent
0.09	728	182	19	1,818	455	48	1,254	139	33
1.02	816	204	21	1,730	433	46	1,254	139	33
1.14	912	228	24	1,634	409	43	1,254	139	33
1.25	1,000	250	26	1,564	387	41	1,254	139	33

FEMALE • Weight: 130 pounds • Target Daily Caloric Intake: 2,340

Protein Level (g/lb)	Protein Composition			Carbohydrate Composition			Fat Composition		
	Calories	Grams	Percent	Calories	Grams	Percent	Calories	Grams	Percent
0.09	473	118	20	1,095	274	47	772	86	33
1.02	532	133	23	1,036	259	44	772	86	33
1.14	591	148	25	977	244	42	772	86	33
1.25	650	163	28	918	229	39	772	86	33

Determining Your Caloric Intake

The starting point for any diet program is quantifying your daily caloric expenditure. Once you know your caloric expenditure, you can then customize your own Nutrient Timing System nutrition program. (We will show you how to do the latter in the next chapter). In Appendix A: Caloric

Expenditure Calculator on page 174, we present a simple do-it-yourself system to determine how many calories you burn in a twenty-four-hour period.

3 + 1—The Secret for Implementing Nutrient Timing

Three plus one is all it takes to get the full benefits of Nutrient Timing— that is, nutrient intervention three times around your workout plus one healthy diet. As shown in Table 7.2, you also have the option of taking another growth phase supplement as a post-dinner snack to achieve greater muscle growth.

Table 7.2 outlines a sample food plan for a 200-pound strength athlete who works out once per day. The goal protein level is 1.1 gram per pound for a daily total of 228 grams. As you can see, it is not a complex program. However, it does require paying special attention to nutrition during the periods when your muscles are most susceptible to damage and when they are most susceptible to growth. This may mean a slight change in your eating habits.

TABLE 7.2. Daily Caloric Composition for a 200-Pound Male Athlete Who Works Out Once Daily

The goal protein amount is 228 grams and the goal caloric intake is 3,800 calories.

	Protein	Carbohydrate	Fat	Calories
Breakfast	28 g	80 g	28 g	684
Workout (Energy Supplement)	6 g	24 g	1 g	129
Postworkout (Anabolic Supplement)	15 g	45 g	1 g	249
2 Hours Postworkout (Growth Supplement)	20 g	4 g	1 g	105
Lunch	46 g	82 g	18 g	674
Snack	14 g	92 g	33 g	721
Dinner	56 g	80 g	49 g	985
Post-dinner (Growth Supplement)	20 g	4 g	1 g	105
TOTAL	**226 g**	**411 g**	**138 g**	**3,790**

In our examples, we have scheduled your workout in the morning. We recognize that with busy schedules athletes do not have a set time each day for their workout. To implement the Nutrient Timing System, you do not have to perform a morning workout. However, whenever your workout occurs, it is important that you consume the proper nutrients during the three critical phases. If need be, adjust your meals accordingly.

Table 7.3 on page 90 summarizes the ideal nutrient composition for each phase of the Nutrient Timing System. As mentioned previously, the ideal form for the NTS supplement in the Energy Phase is a beverage, which will help replace fluids lost during your workout. Although there are many advantages to consuming a beverage for the Anabolic and Growth Phase, solid food can work just as well as long as the nutrient composition is optimal. In the next chapter, one of the country's leading nutritionists, Dr. Susan Kleiner, author of *Power Eating*, will show you how to create your own NTS nutrition program.

KEY TAKEAWAYS

- A high-protein diet consisting of 41 to 48 percent carbohydrate, 19 to 26 percent protein, and 33 percent fat is an excellent one for strength athletes.

- 41 to 48 percent carbohydrate and 33 percent fat will give you the necessary energy for a strong workout and maintaining a healthy immune system.

- 3 + 1 is the secret for implementing Nutrient Timing effectively: three nutrient interventions during and after workouts plus one healthy diet.

TABLE 7.3. NTS Recommended Supplements Nutrient Profile

NTS PHASE		NTS Objective	Nutrient	Amount
ENERGY PHASE 10 minutes prior to and during a workout		• Increase nutrient delivery to muscles and spare muscle glycogen and protein	High-glycemic carbohydrates (glucose, sucrose, and maltodextrin)	20–26 g
		• Limit immune system suppression	Whey protein	5–6 g
			Leucine	1 g
		• Minimize muscle damage	Vitamin C	30–120 mg
			Vitamin E	20–60 IU
		• Set the nutritional stage for a faster recovery following your workout	Sodium	100–250 IU
			Potassium	60–120 mg
			Magnesium	60–120 mg
ANABOLIC PHASE Within 45 minutes after a workout		• Shift metabolic machinery from a catabolic state to an anabolic state	Whey protein	13–15 g
		• Speed the elimination of metabolic wastes by increasing muscle blood flow	High-glycemic carbohydrates (glucose, sucrose, and maltodextrin)	40–50 g
			Leucine	1–2 g
		• Replenish muscle glycogen stores	Glutamine	1–2 g
		• Initiate tissue repair and set the stage for muscle growth	Vitamin C	60–120 mg
		• Reduce muscle damage and bolster the immune system	Vitamin E	80–400 IU
GROWTH PHASE	**Rapid Segment** The first 4 hours after a workout	• Maintain increased insulin sensitivity	Whey protein	14 g
		• Maintain the anabolic state	Casein	2 g
			Leucine	3 g
	Sustained Segment The next 16–18 hours after a workout	• Maintain positive nitrogen balance and stimulate protein synthesis	Glutamine	1 g
		• Promote protein turnover and muscle development	High-glycemic carbohydrates	2–4 g

The NTS
Nutrition Program

Susan Kleiner, Ph.D., R.D., F.A.C.N., C.N.S.

Now that NTS has shown you why your body needs the right combination of nutrients at the right times to promote maximum energy, recovery and growth, you must learn to translate the scientific facts into food. What, how much, and when should you eat to stay healthy and get the results that you want?

Think of this chapter as both a simple and detailed outline of your menu plan. If you're merely seeking the basic facts to get started, then the simple menu templates and sample food menus provided here are the best places to begin. But if you're interested in learning all the details, you'll find them in this chapter as well.

NTS FOOD GROUPS

The easiest way to categorize foods is to put them into groups according to their common nutrients. Using food groups helps to ensure that a diet is designed with the variety of nutrients required to promote energy metabolism, tissue growth and repair, and lifetime health. The Nutrient Timing System uses the specific food groups shown in Table 8.1. This table segments food into twelve groups. You may notice a few tweaks from the traditional food groups outlined in the well-known USDA Food Guide Pyramid.

To make it easy for you to substitute one food item for another in a specific food group, each group item listed has an equivalent nutrient composition and the same number of calories. For example, under the starch group, one slice of bread is equivalent to a half cup of cooked pasta.

Creating Your Personal NTS Nutrition Plan

Step 1

Determine your daily caloric intake using the Caloric Expenditure Calculator in Appendix A on page 174.

Step 2

Select the meal plan templates provided in Appendix B on page 177 that are closest to your calorie needs. The meal plan templates are designed to deliver a daily protein content of 1.14 grams of protein per pound of body weight.

Step 3

Refer to Table 8.1 to personalize your diet. Select real foods from this table and fill them into the templates.

If your calorie needs are slightly different from those listed in the templates, do the following:

Step 1

Determine your daily caloric intake using the Caloric Expenditure Calculator in Appendix A on page 174.

Step 2

Distribute your calories as follows: 24 percent protein, 43 percent carbohydrate, and 33 percent fat.

Step 3

Adjust the protein, carbohydrate, and fat percentages in the template by adding or subtracting foods according to their individual nutrient contents listed in Table 8.1. Select foods from this table to personalize your diet.

Except when noted, the templates are designed for an individual who works out once a day. If you work out twice a day, add a second round of Energy, Anabolic, and Growth Phase supplements to sufficiently adjust your caloric intake.

TABLE 8.1. NTS Food and Supplement Group

Food/ Supplement Group	Item Substitution/Serving Size	Nutrient Composition			
		Protein	Carbs	Fat	Calories
Starch	1 slice bread; $^1/_2$ cup cooked cereal, pasta, or starch vegetable; 1 medium potato; $^1/_2$ cup rice; 1 ounce whole-grain ready-to-eat cereal; $^1/_2$ bun, bagel, or English muffin; 1 small roll; 3–4 small or 2 large crackers	3 g	15 g	1 g	81
Fruit	1 small to medium fresh fruit, $^1/_2$ cup canned or fresh fruit, or $^1/_2$ cup fruit juice; $^1/_4$ cup of dried fruit; $^1/_2$ grapefruit; 1 melon wedge	—	15 g	—	60
Milk	1 cup fat-free or up to 2-percent reduced-fat milk or soy milk	8 g	12 g	1 g	89
Added Sugars	These foods contain only sugar and are counted by teaspoons of added sugar. If, for example, the cereal or yogurt you select contains added sugar, the sugar must be accounted for in your diet.	—	4 g	—	16
Vegetables	$^1/_2$ cup cooked vegetables or vegetable juice; 1 cup raw vegetables.	2 g	5 g	—	28
Meat/Meat Substitutes	1 ounce beef, fish, poultry, or cheese; $^1/_2$ cup beans, peas, or lentils (count legumes as 1 starch plus 1 very lean meat)				
Very Lean Choices	White-meat skinless poultry; cod, flounder, haddock, halibut, or trout; tuna fresh or canned in water; all shellfish; cheese with 1 gram or less fat per ounce; processed sandwich meats with 1 gram or less fat per ounce; egg whites	7 g	—	—	28
Lean Choices	USDA Select or Choice grades of lean beef, pork, lamb, or veal, trimmed of fat; dark-meat skinless poultry or white meat chicken with skin; oysters, salmon, catfish, sardines, or tuna canned in oil; 4.5% cottage cheese with 3 grams or less fat per ounce ($^1/_4$ cup); processed sandwich meat with 3 grams or less fat per ounce	7 g	—	3 g	55

Food/ Supplement Group	Item Substitution/ Serving Size	Nutrient Composition			
		Protein	Carbs	Fat	Calories
Medium-Fat Choices	Most styles of beef, pork, lamb, veal, trimmed of fat; prime grades trimmed of fat; dark-meat chicken with skin, or ground turkey or ground chicken; any fresh or canned fish product not breaded or fried; cheese with 5 grams or less fat per ounce; whole egg; soy milk (1 cup); tempeh ($\frac{1}{4}$ cup); tofu (4 oz or $\frac{1}{2}$ cup)	7 g	—	5 g	73
Fat	1 tsp butter, margarine, or vegetable oil; 1 tbsp regular salad dressing; 2 tbsp reduced-fat salad dressing; 1 tbsp reduced-fat mayonnaise; 2 tbsp reduced-fat cream cheese; $\frac{1}{8}$ medium avocado; 8 olives; 6–10 nuts; 2 tsp peanut butter or tahini; 1 tbsp seeds, or 1–2 tbsp ground seeds. 6 ounces of regular beer or wine, or 8 ounces of light beer is equivalent to 2 fat servings	—	—	5 g	45
NTS Energy Supplement	High-glycemic carbohydrate and (protein 4 g carb to 1 g protein ratio) plus leucine, vitamin C, and vitamin E (in form of beverage to replace fluid lost during workout)	6 g	24 g	1 g	129
NTS Anabolic Supplement	High-glycemic carbohydrate and protein (3 g carb to 1 g protein ratio) plus glutamine, leucine, vitamin C, and vitamin E (in form of solid food or beverage)	15 g	45 g	1 g	249
NTS Growth Supplement	Protein and high-glycemic carbohydrates (5 g protein to 1 g carb ratio) plus glutamine, leucine, vitamin C, and vitamin E (in form of solid food or beverage)	20 g	4 g	1 g	105

Review the food groups to become familiar with how different foods are categorized. Next, turn to the Daily Food Group Templates in tables 8.2, 8.3, and 8.4 on pages 96–98. We've designed the following three templates with menus:

- **Profile A:** 200-pound male who works out once a day

- **Profile B:** 200-pound male who works out twice a day

- **Profile C:** 130-pound female who works out once a day

The Daily Food Group Templates are an overview of what you need to eat and when to eat it using the Nutrient Timing System. Thereafter, look at the sample food menus for each profile in Tables 8.5, 8.6, and 8.7 on pages 99–104. Based on the Daily Food Group Templates, we provide a sample NTS Food Menu Plan by placing specific food choices in place of the food groups listed in the template. For example, you'll see "1 milk" in the template replaced by "1 cup nonfat milk" in the Food Menu Plan. You'll see "2 starch" in the template replaced by "1 medium baked potato and ⅓ cup brown rice" in the Food Menu Plan. By using the Daily Food Group Template, you can personalize your diet by choosing the foods you like from each food group. It's that easy to design your own individualized Nutrient Timing System Nutrition Plan.

Every detail has been figured into these plans. The combinations of foods have been designed to maximize your training. You don't need to add anything with one very important exception: water. In addition to the many beverages used in the meal plans, your body needs at least 40–48 ounces of water per day. You can drink water with your meals and snacks as long as it doesn't hamper your appetite. If you find that you fill up with water during a meal and can't finish your food, then drink water between meals and snacks.

DAILY FOOD GROUP TEMPLATES

PROFILE A

Male • **Weight:** 200 pounds

Energy: 19 calories per pound

Workout Regimen: Once daily

Goal Daily Caloric Needs: 3,800 calories

Protein Level: 1.14 grams protein per pound of body weight

TABLE 8.2. Daily Food Group Template for Profile A				
	Servings	**Protein**	**Carbohydrates**	**Fat**	**Calories**
Starch	8	24 g	120 g	8 g	648
Fruit	8	—	120 g	—	480
Milk	3	24 g	36 g	3 g	267
Added Sugars	7	—	28 g	—	112
Vegetables	6	12 g	30 g	—	168
Meat/Meat Substitutes					
Very Lean	7	49	—	—	196
Lean	6	42 g	—	18 g	330
Medium Fat	2	14 g	—	10 g	146
Fat	19	—	—	95 g	855
NTS Energy Supplement	1	6 g	24 g	1 g	129
NTS Anabolic Supplement	1	15 g	45 g	1 g	249
NTS Growth Supplement	2	40 g	8 g	2 g	210
Total Grams		226 g	411 g	138 g	
Daily Calories (actual)		904	1,644	1,242	3,790
Nutrient Composition		24%	43%	33%	

PROFILE B

Male • **Weight:** 200 pounds

Energy: 21 calories per pound

Workout Regimen: Twice daily

Goal Daily Caloric Needs: 4,200 calories

Protein Level: 1.24 grams protein per pound of body weight

TABLE 8.3. Daily Food Group Template for Profile B

	Servings	Protein	Carbohydrates	Fat	Calories
Starch	8	24 g	120 g	8 g	648
Fruit	7	–	105 g	–	420
Milk	4	32 g	48 g	4 g	356
Added Sugars	3	–	12 g	–	48
Vegetables	6	12 g	30 g	–	168
Meat/Meat Substitutes					
Very Lean	6	42 g	–	–	168
Lean	4	28 g	–	12 g	220
Medium Fat	4	28 g	–	20 g	292
Fat	20	–	–	100 g	900
NTS Energy Supplement	2	12 g	48 g	2 g	258
NTS Anabolic Supplement	2	30 g	90 g	2 g	498
NTS Growth Supplement	2	40 g	8 g	2 g	210
Total Grams		248 g	461 g	150 g	
Daily Calories (actual)		992	1,844	1,350	4,186
Nutrient Composition		24%	44%	32%	

PROFILE C

Female • Weight: 130 pounds

Energy: 18 calories per pound

Workout Regimen: Once daily

Goal Daily Caloric Needs: 2,340 calories

Protein Level: 1.1 grams protein per pound of body weight

TABLE 8.4. Daily Food Group Templates for Profile C					
	Servings	Protein	Carbohydrates	Fat	Calories
Starch	3	9 g	45 g	3 g	243
Fruit	5	—	75 g	—	300
Milk	2	16 g	24 g	2 g	178
Added Sugars	2	—	8 g	—	32
Vegetables	5	10 g	25 g	—	140
Meat/Meat Substitutes					
Very Lean	3	21 g	—	—	84
Lean	3	21 g	—	9 g	165
Medium Fat	3	21 g	—	15 g	219
Fat	11	—	—	55 g	495
NTS Energy Supplement	1	6 g	24 g	1 g	129
NTS Anabolic Supplement	1	15 g	45 g	1 g	249
NTS Growth Supplement	1	20 g	4 g	1 g	105
Total Grams		139 g	250 g	87 g	
Daily Calories (actual)		556	1,000	783	2,339
Nutrient Composition		24%	43%	33%	

TABLE 8.5. Sample Food Menu Plan for Profile A

	Food Group	Servings	Menu Item	Protein	Carb	Fat	Cal
Breakfast	Starch	2	2 slices whole-grain toast	6	30	2	162
	Fruit	2	1 cup orange juice	—	30	—	120
	Milk	1	1 cup milk	8	12	1	89
	Added Sugars	2	2 tsp 100% fruit spread	—	8	—	32
	Med Fat	2	2 whole eggs	14	—	10	146
	Fat	3	2 tsp butter, 2 tbsp cream	—	—	15	135
Breakfast Total				28	80	28	684
Workout	NTS Energy Supplement	1		6	24	1	129
Immediately Postworkout	NTS Anabolic Supplement	1		15	45	1	249
2 Hours Postworkout	NTS Growth Supplement	1		20	4	1	105
Lunch	Starch	2	2 slices whole wheat or rye	6	30	2	162
	Fruit	2	1 cup fresh fruit cup	—	30	—	120
	Milk	1	1 cup milk	8	12	1	89
	Vegetables	2	lettuce & tomato, tossed salad	4	10	—	56
	Very Lean	4	4 oz sliced turkey	28	—	—	112
	Fat	3	1 tbsp reduced-fat or 1 tsp regular mayo + 4 tbsp reduced-fat or 2 tbsp regular salad dressing	—	—	15	135
Lunch Total				46	82	18	674

	Food Group	Servings	Menu Item	Protein	Carb	Fat	Cal
Snack	Starch	2	2 slices whole-grain bread	6	30	2	162
	Fruit	2	I cup grapes	—	30	—	120
	Milk	I	I cup milk	8	12	I	89
	Added Sugars	5	2 tbsp 100% fruit spread	—	20	—	80
	Fat	6	3 tbsp natural peanut butter	—	—	30	270
Snack Total				14	92	33	721
Dinner	Starch	2	I medium baked potato + $\frac{1}{3}$ cup brown rice	6	30	2	162
	Fruit	2	$\frac{2}{3}$ cup cranberry juice cocktail	—	15	—	120
	Vegetables	4	I cup asparagus, tossed salad	8	20	—	112
	Very Lean	3	3 oz shrimp cocktail	21	—	—	84
	Lean	6	6 oz salmon	42	—	18	330
	Fat	7	2 tbsp sour cream, I tsp flax oil, 3 tsp olive oil, $\frac{1}{4}$ avocado	—	—	35	315
Dinner Total				56	65	49	957
Post Dinner	NTS Growth Supplement	I		28	5	I	141
GRAND TOTAL				226	411	138	3,790

TABLE 8.6. Food Menu Plan for Profile B

	Food Group	Servings	Menu Item	Protein	Carb	Fat	Cal
Breakfast	Starch	2	2 slices whole-grain bread	6	30	2	162
	Fruit	2	I cup orange juice	—	30	—	120
	Milk	I	I cup milk	8	12	I	89
	Added Sugars	I	I tsp sugar	—	4	—	16
	Very Lean	2	4 egg whites	14	—	—	56
	Med Fat	2	2 whole eggs	14	—	10	146
	Fat	3	2 tsp butter, 2 tbsp cream	—	—	15	135
Breakfast Total				42	76	28	724
Workout	NTS Energy Supplement	I		6	24	I	129
Immediately Postworkout	NTS Anabolic Supplement	I		15	45	I	249
2 Hours Postworkout	NTS Growth Supplement	I		20	4	I	105
Lunch	Starch	2	2 slices whole-wheat or rye bread	6	30	2	162
	Fruit	2	I cup fresh fruit	—	30	—	120
	Vegetables	2	lettuce and tomato, tossed salad	4	10	—	56
	Very Lean	2	2 oz turkey	14	—	—	56
	Med Fat	2	2 oz mozzarella cheese	14	—	10	146
	Fat	5	I tbsp reduced-fat or I tsp regular mayo, 3 tbsp regular dressing or 6 tbsp reduced-fat dressing	—	—	20	180
Lunch Total				46	82	33	809

	Food Group	Servings	Menu Item	Protein	Carb	Fat	Cal
Workout	NTS Energy Supplement	1		6	24	1	129
Immediately Postworkout	NTS Anabolic Supplement	1		15	45	1	249
2 Hours Postworkout	NTS Growth Supplement	1		20	4	1	105
Dinner	Starch	1	1 med baked potato	3	15	1	81
	Fruit	3	1 cup cranberry juice cocktail, 1 melon wedge	—	45	—	180
	Vegetables	4	1 cup asparagus, tossed salad	8	20	—	112
	Very Lean	1	1 oz salad shrimp	7	—	—	28
	Lean	4	4 oz salmon	28	—	12	220
	Fat	7	1 tbsp sour cream, 1 tsp flax oil, 2 tsp olive oil, 1/4 avocado	—	—	35	315
Dinner Total				46	80	48	936
Snack	Starch	2	2 slices whole-wheat bread	6	30	2	162
	Fruit	2	1 cup grapes	—	30	—	120
	Milk	1	1 cup milk	8	12	1	89
	Added Sugars	5	1.5 tbsp 100% fruit spread	—	20	—	80
	Vegetables	1	carrot and celery sticks	2	5	—	28
	Fat	6	3 tbsp natural peanut butter	—	—	30	270
Snack Total				16	97	33	749
GRAND TOTAL				248	461	150	4,186

Table 8.7. Food Menu Plan for Profile C

	Food Group	Servings	Menu Item	Protein	Carb	Fat	Cal
Breakfast	Starch	1	1/2 cup shredded wheat cereal	3	15	1	81
	Fruit	2	3/4 cup blueberries, 1/2 cup orange juice		30		120
	Milk	1	1 cup milk	8	12	1	89
	Fat	1	1–2 tbsp ground flaxseed			5	45
Breakfast Total				11	57	7	335
Workout	NTS Energy Supplement	1		6	24	1	129
Immediately Postworkout	NTS Anabolic Supplement	1		15	45	1	249
2 Hours Postworkout	NTS Growth Supplement	1		20	4	1	105
Lunch	Starch	1	1 whole grain roll	3	15	1	81
	Fruit	2	1 cup fresh fruit cup		30		120
	Vegetables	2	large tossed salad	4	10		56
	Med Fat	3	1 hard boiled egg, 2 oz mozzarella cheese	21		15	219
	Fat	3	4 tbsp reduced-fat or 2 tbsp regular salad dressing, 1/8 avocado			15	135
Lunch Total				28	55	31	611
Snack	Milk	1	1 cup plain yogurt	8	12	1	89
	Added Sugars	2	2 tsp honey		8		32
	Fat	3	handful (18) almonds & cashews			15	135
Snack Total				8	20	16	256

	Food Group	Servings	Menu Item	Protein	Carb	Fat	Cal
Dinner	Starch	1	1 med baked potato	3	15	1	81
	Fruit	1	1 cup fresh raspberries		15		60
	Vegetables	3	1 cup asparagus, tossed salad	6	15		84
	Very Lean	3	3 oz salad shrimp or shrimp cocktail	21			84
	Lean	3	3 oz salmon	21		9	165
	Fat	4	1 tbsp sour cream, 2 tsp olive oil, 2 tbsp reduced-fat or 1 tbsp regular salad dressing			20	180
Dinner Total				51	45	30	654
GRAND TOTAL				139	250	87	2,339

Experiment with various strategies to find which one or which combination of strategies works in your life. You might find that copying the template and carrying it around with you is helpful. You can pull it out when you're shopping for groceries or ordering at a restaurant. Alternatively, you can develop your own seven-day menu plan and shop and prepare your food accordingly. Most people find that some combination of these two strategies works best.

The key to success is planning ahead. Although we've done the hard part of designing the program for you, you will still have to shop and prepare your meals, and follow your template when ordering at a restaurant. But you don't have to get neurotic about this. The goal is to follow these plans on a regular basis. If you have been invited to a dinner party or are traveling and just can't quite meet the template guidelines, don't sweat it. Use the supplements to fuel yourself around your exercise, and do your best to make good choices the rest of the day. As long as you follow the plan on a usual basis, what happens on the unusual days will have little impact.

FOOD CHOICES: WHAT TO BUY?

When you get to the supermarket, what should you buy? What are the good food choices? It's not surprising that the foods that promote health and prevent disease are the same foods that maximize energy and growth.

Plant foods will be the mainstay of your diet. They are full of vitamins, minerals, phytochemicals, carbohydrates, and fibers that are essential for energy, growth, and health. Choose whole, unprocessed fruits, vegetables, grains, beans, nuts, and seeds as frequently as possible. Vegetable oils and 100 percent fruit juices also play important roles in your diet. Variety within each of the food groups is just as essential as choosing foods representing each food group. For instance, eat carrots, broccoli, asparagus, cucumber, lettuce, and tomato, instead of eating solely from the bag of mini-carrots that you have stashed in your refrigerator for every meal.

Excellent sources of protein are lean cuts of beef, fish, poultry, eggs, and nonfat and low-fat dairy and soy products. Nonfat and low-fat dairy products are ideal sources of all the bone-building nutrients, some of which are also important for energy and protein metabolism. Again, variety is very important here. Different protein foods offer a mixture of different nutrients in addition to protein. Fatty fish like salmon are high in omega-3 fats, eggs are high in lecithin, dairy is high in calcium, and soy is high in isoflavones and fiber.

Shop the perimeter of your supermarket. That's where you'll find the butcher/fishmonger, fresh bakery, produce, and dairy sections. The aisles that offer canned beans and nuts are also important. Generally, the further you progress toward the center of the store, the more processed and refined the food becomes.

Highly refined foods are not only depleted of the nutrients through heavy processing, but they are usually also very high in added sugar. While sugar can be a friend to an athlete when used around exercise according to the Nutrient Timing System, sugar at other times of the day amounts to empty, nonfunctional calories. The Nutrient Timing menu plans are designed to optimize added sugar in the diet to enhance both taste and performance. Sugar is added to the menus in teaspoons with exercise timing in mind. Because your body will benefit most from the timing strategy designed into the menus, it is best to follow that strategy most frequently. But if you would like to have all your added teaspoons of sugar at one meal, it will not hinder your progress if you restrict it to special occasions.

Are High-Protein Diets and Protein Supplements Dangerous?

John M. Berardi, C.S.C.S.

You may have heard the rumors, the recommendations of dietitians, and the firm disapproval of medical professionals. They say that those protein supplements will "destroy your kidneys," "cause dehydration," and "ruin your bones." But you've also heard a number of other experts, backed up by clinical trials, telling you there's no danger. So what's the truth? Are protein supplements dangerous? Well, let's take a look at the research.

Is There Impaired Kidney Function?

Although studies have been published showing that in individuals with unhealthy kidneys, excessive protein intake could place undue strain on the kidneys, healthy individuals have little to worry about with high-protein diets. To demonstrate this, a recent study showed that when bodybuilders consumed up to 1.3 grams of protein per pound (2.8 g/kg) of body weight, kidney function was not impaired. In fact, in an older study conducted with female rats, kidney function seemed to be improved with high-protein diets.

What About Calcium Loss?

A few original studies demonstrated that when protein intake was raised to 140–225 grams per day, excess calcium was lost from the urine at a faster rate than normal. However, in these studies, calcium intake as well as phosphorus intake was restricted and not allowed to increase in proportion to the protein intake. Since whole-food protein sources contain both calcium and phosphorus and even protein supplements are fortified with calcium and phosphorus, it only makes sense that increases in protein intake are typically accompanied by increased dietary calcium and phosphorus. In this context, the research has demonstrated that consuming additional protein results in a positive calcium balance and there are no adverse affects on bone calcium content.

Will You Experience Dehydration?

It's true that lots of extra protein can cause extra water excretion (that is, more frequent urination). But alcohol and coffee do the same thing. An easy solution is to drink a few extra glasses of water per day. It will help stave off dehydration and assist other metabolic processes as well. The relationship between water loss and high-protein diets has been observed in nonathletes. The study conducted with marine recruits discussed in Chapter 5 suggests that this may not be a problem during exercise. In the marine-recruit study, there was a dramatic decline in the incidence of dehydration in subjects taking the carbohydrate/protein drink versus those consuming water or carbohydrate and water. The 83 percent decrease in heat exhaustion in the carbohydrate/protein group may be explained by the lower lean body mass of the subjects who did not suffer heat exhaustion or by the fact that the increased protein resulted in higher blood levels of a specific protein, which reduced water loss.

What about Constipation?

Nutritionists and dietitians claim that diets high in protein are low in fiber. Insufficient bulk in the digestive system can cause constipation. However, this problem can be easily remedied. Simply choose the right foods such as fibrous vegetables and starchy breads and pasta, and drink sufficient amounts of water.

From this information, it should be clear that the "dangers" of a high-protein diet and protein supplements are overstated. There is no question that athletes benefit from a higher protein intake. As there are no clear risks associated with them, protein supplements can provide a convenient and safe way to get extra protein in the diet.

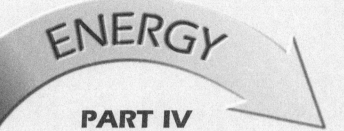

ENERGY

GROWTH

ANABOLIC

PART IV

*NUTRITION
AND
PERFORMANCE*

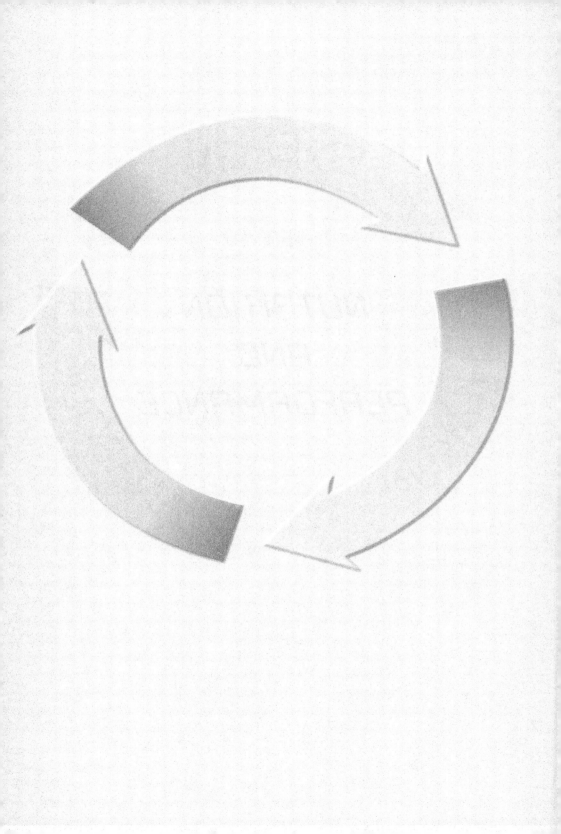

Nutrient Activators
and Sports Supplements

Nutrient activation takes place when one nutrient helps another nutrient perform its job more efficiently. More exactly, nutrient activation is a process by which the biological effects of a certain nutrient are influenced through direct or indirect interaction with one or more other nutrients. This is a key concept in the Nutrient Timing System.

As you've learned, muscle recovery and growth occur fastest when the right nutrients are consumed at the right times in relation to training. That's simple enough, but it's also important to understand how these various nutrients interact to promote muscle growth. This chapter discusses the key nutrient activators and their potential benefits to the body when taken at the right time. It also alerts you to the questionable activators—supplements you might be taking to enhance your performance that just might not work the way they are purported to.

NUTRIENT ACTIVATORS

Most strength athletes think of nutrients in terms of their direct effects not in terms of their indirect effects. For example, they think of protein as the constituent that muscles are made of, but they don't think of protein as a nutrient that can enhance muscle glycogen storage by stimulating insulin (protein as activator). Let's take a look at the important nutrient activators that can cooperate to maximize the rate at which proteins become biologically active components of your growing muscles.

Carbohydrate

The most important nutrient activator in relation to protein is carbohydrate. This connection is mediated through insulin, which is strongly stimulated by the consumption of carbohydrate. Insulin not only stimulates the transport of amino acids into the muscle, but also activates key elements of the protein synthetic machinery. The manner in which amino acids activate protein synthesis is different from the manner in which insulin does, so their effects on protein synthesis become additive. Insulin also helps decrease protein degradation, which is important for tipping the protein turnover balance toward net protein accretion (an increase in the protein concentration within the muscle). So, in order to get greater protein synthesis, you need to consume carbohydrate along with your protein drink during the Anabolic and Growth phases. For example, researchers have shown that a combined protein/carbohydrate supplement taken after exercise results in a 38 percent faster rate of protein synthesis as a protein supplement without carbohydrate. It is therefore fair to say that the path to greater protein synthesis and ultimately to muscle development is traveled quicker when carbohydrate is consumed with protein.

Protein

Just as carbohydrate activates protein, protein is able to work with carbohydrate to activate certain metabolic processes, which include muscle glucose uptake and glycogen storage. As mentioned, one effect of combined carbohydrate/protein supplementation is a greater insulin response. Protein alone has only a small effect on blood insulin levels. However, when protein is combined with carbohydrate, the insulin response is greater than that produced by either carbohydrate or protein alone.

Insulin is, as we've seen, a strong activator of muscle glucose uptake and glycogen synthesis. However, the nutrient activation caused by protein is not due solely to a greater insulin response. Certain amino acids such as leucine and isoleucine can activate muscle glucose uptake and glycogen storage through insulin-independent pathways. Thus, the addition of protein to a carbohydrate supplement can greatly increase the rate of muscle glycogen synthesis. In research studies, the addition of protein to a carbohydrate supplement has been shown to increase glycogen storage by 40 to 100 percent during the early hours of postworkout recovery.

Amino Acids

Amino acids are a broad class of structurally similar biochemical compounds that serve as the building blocks of protein. As parts of a protein molecule, they are linked together by peptide bonds. Thousands of amino acids can be linked to form proteins involved in cell structure (membranes), cell function (actin and myosin), or energy production (myosin ATPase). In addition, amino acids can function as biochemical messengers and as intermediates in metabolism. Three amino acids in particular are important nutrient activators in NTS: arginine, glutamine, and leucine.

ARGININE

Arginine is important in helping the muscles to manufacture other amino acids. In addition, arginine is an excellent stimulator of insulin and therefore has the ability to enhance carbohydrate metabolism.

Another beneficial characteristic of arginine is its ability to increase blood flow. When blood vessels are expanded (or dilated), greater blood flow is possible. This is particularly important during exercise and recovery from exercise, because at these times muscles need greater amounts of oxygen and nutrients and there is also a greater need to remove metabolic byproducts such as carbon dioxide and lactic acid. An essential regulator of vasodilation is nitric oxide (NO). The production of NO requires arginine, which serves as a precursor for NO formation. Arginine supplementation has been shown to stimulate the NO system. A number of arginine supplements are now sold as circulation boosters. There is, however, a downside to supplementing with this amino acid: consuming arginine in large amounts (greater than 10 grams) can cause gastrointestinal distress.

GLUTAMINE

Glutamine is the most abundant amino acid in the blood and muscle cells. It comprises more than 60 percent of the free amino acid pool in muscle tissue. Glutamine is also the most nitrogen-rich amino acid, supplying 35 percent of the nitrogen that muscle cells use to synthesize proteins.

Glutamine is considered to be a "conditionally essential" amino acid because, although the body can synthesize it, there are times when the body's high demand for glutamine exceeds its glutamine stores and manufacturing efforts. Several kinds of stress can dramatically increase the body's glutamine needs. Strenuous exercise, injuries, and illnesses are the main ones.

In addition to promoting protein synthesis, glutamine, by helping to maintain a positive nitrogen balance in muscle tissue, also prevents protein breakdown, which is equally important when it comes to building muscle.

At one time it was believed that carbohydrate provided all of the necessary nutrition to support immune system function. It is now well documented that glutamine is also an important nutrient for cells of the immune system. During prolonged exercise, glutamine levels are depleted. Within twenty-four hours, glutamine levels usually return to normal, assuming the athlete is consuming a healthy diet. However, in athletes who train intensively, glutamine levels may be chronically low. Because of the relationship between glutamine and immune system function, these athletes may be more susceptible to upper respiratory tract infections. One study reported that 73 percent of athletes with infection had glutamine levels below normal. This suggests that athletes who train intensively would benefit from glutamine supplementation. Researchers have demonstrated that supplementation could increase baseline levels of glutamine. It has also been demonstrated that when protein is taken following exercise, the normal drop in glutamine can be prevented.

Recent research suggests that glutamine may also promote protein synthesis by activating metabolic pathways through cell volumization (hydration of cells). Protein synthesis proceeds more quickly when muscle fibers are enlarged or swollen. Glutamine draws water and salt into muscle cells, thereby expediting protein synthesis.

Finally, glutamine can also promote the storage of glycogen. In a study by Bowtell and colleagues from the University of Dundee, Scotland, groups of six subjects each cycled until exhausted and were then given either a carbohydrate supplement, a glutamine supplement, or a carbohydrate/glutamine supplement. Although the carbohydrate/glutamine supplement did not promote more muscle glycogen storage than the carbohydrate supplement, it was more effective in increasing the liver glycogen stores.

Studies have shown that a minimum of 2 grams of glutamine is needed to increase plasma growth hormone levels. An 8-gram dose has been demonstrated to be effective in promoting glycogen resynthesis. Because of glutamine's role in supporting the immune system and postexercise muscle recovery, it should be a standard part of a postexercise meal.

Studies have shown that short- and long-term glutamine supplementation is safe in humans. Oral doses of glutamine as high as 0.3 grams per kilogram of body weight have been administered with no evidence of toxicity.

Table 9.1 lists the glutamine content for a variety of foods.

TABLE 9.1. Glutamine Content of Selected Food	
Food	**Content**
Round steak (3 ounces)	4.05 g
Chicken breast (3 ounces)	3.74 g
Chicken thigh (3 ounces)	3.31 g
Ground beef (3 ounces)	3.19 g
Ham (3 ounces)	2.68 g
Sole/flounder fillet (3 ounces)	2.39 g
Skim milk (1 cup)	1.67 g
Mozzarella cheese (1 ounce)	1.65 g
Cheddar cheese (1 ounce)	1.59 g
Dry roasted peanuts (1 ounce)	1.40 g
Lentils ($^1/_2$ cup)	1.39 g
Soy milk ($^1/_2$ cup)	1.35 g
Black beans ($^1/_2$ cup)	1.16 g
Large boiled egg (1 large)	0.82 g

BRANCHED-CHAIN AMINO ACIDS (BCAAS)

Leucine, isoleucine, and valine are three special amino acids known as the branched-chain amino acids (BCAAs). They serve as precursors for the synthesis of glutamine and alanine, two amino acids that are used up rapidly and in large quantities during intense exercise. Isoleucine and valine are used as a direct source of energy during exercise. Ingestion of BCAAs during exercise not only provides needed energy but may also prevent muscle protein breakdown, resulting in faster postworkout recovery.

In one study, Coombes and McNaughton had two groups of subjects exercise for two hours on a stationary bicycle. One group had taken a daily BCAA supplement for the preceding fourteen days, while the second group had received a placebo. In both groups, biomarkers of muscle damage were elevated from four hours to five days after cycling. However, this indication of muscle damage was substantially lower in the BCAA group.

Leucine in particular is one of the most potent nutrient activators in relation to muscle growth. Leucine is not just used as a building block for muscle proteins, but it can also help amplify muscle protein synthesis. First, it can increase blood insulin levels by stimulating the release of insulin from the pancreas. Second, it can work cooperatively with insulin to initiate protein synthesis. Insulin serves to activate the signal pathway, while leucine enhances the signal for protein synthesis at the level of peptide initiation (translation). This effect is particularly pronounced after exercise, when the muscle cells exhibit increased insulin sensitivity. Some research also suggests that leucine is able to stimulate both muscle protein synthesis and glucose uptake through another insulin-independent mechanism.

Creatine

Creatine is the most popular muscle-building nutritional supplement. In the early 1990s, creatine exploded in popularity among athletes in strength and speed sports when research demonstrated that creatine supplementation could increase the strength and muscle mass gains associated with resistance training.

Creatine is necessary for the production of creatine phosphate (CP), the high-energy phosphate compound stored in the muscles and responsible for the rapid resynthesis of ATP. Creatine can be manufactured from its constituent amino acids in the liver and through dietary consumption of creatine, which is found in animal foods such as beef. Creatine supplementation can significantly increase the amount of creatine that is stored in the muscles and thereby increase CP stores.

Many studies have demonstrated that creatine supplementation will enhance training-induced gains in muscle strength and mass. For example, in a study conducted by Vandenberghe and colleagues, subjects were placed on creatine or placebo throughout a ten-week strength-training program. Compared with placebo, maximal strength was increased by 20 to 25 percent and muscle mass by 60 percent with creatine supplementation. Also, Kreider and colleagues reported that college football players who supplemented with creatine and glucose during twenty-eight days of conditioning had greater gains in body weight, muscle mass, and strength compared with players who received a placebo.

Three different mechanisms have been hypothesized to explain how creatine increases muscle mass and strength. The first is that an increase in

CP directly stimulates protein synthesis. The second is that an increase in total muscle creatine draws water into the muscle fiber, causing it to swell, and the swelling then stimulates protein synthesis. The third is that high levels of intramuscular creatine slow the use of ATP during exercise and speeds the recovery of CP. This allows for a harder workout and thus a greater stimulus for protein synthesis.

Most of the studies have utilized a brief loading phase, which is 20 grams per day (4 doses of 5 grams each consumed over the day) for five to seven days. This should increase your skeletal muscles' creatine and CP levels. A maintenance dose of 2.5–5 grams per day should be enough to maintain skeletal muscle creatine and CP levels. Stout and colleagues have shown that the addition of carbohydrate can augment intramuscular creatine, CP, and total creatine levels. A serving of 36 grams of carbohydrate with 5 grams of creatine will improve performance more than creatine alone. However, many athletes often use lower levels of carbohydrate mixed with creatine with good results.

Caffeine

For decades, athletes of all kinds have used the stimulant caffeine—sometimes referred to as the world's most popular drug—to enhance performance. The popularity of caffeine as a performance aid started to rise more than twenty-five years ago when Dr. David Costill of Ball State University reported that caffeine could improve endurance performance. The improvement was thought to be due to caffeine's ability to increase fat oxidation and spare the use of muscle glycogen. While this is still a possible explanation, recent research suggests that caffeine may also delay fatigue by reducing the athlete's perception of effort. Laurent and colleagues found that caffeine increased the concentration of hormone-like substances in the brain called ß-endorphins during exercise. The endorphins affect mood state, reduce perception of pain, and create a sense of well-being.

Caffeine has also been found to delay fatigue during exercise by blocking adenosine receptors. Adenosine is produced during exercise and inhibits the release of the brain neurotransmitter dopamine. Decreases in dopamine, along with increases in serotonin, another brain neurotransmitter have been linked to central nervous system fatigue during exercise. A decrease in the dopamine-serotonin ratio has been shown to reduce arousal, induce sleep, and suppress spontaneous activity of animals.

Caffeine has also been popular among strength athletes because of its metabolic and central nervous system effects. Because caffeine increases fat breakdown and oxidation during exercise, strength athletes have used caffeine to lower body-fat content. In addition, they have used caffeine to increase workout intensity because of its ability to increase arousal and reduce perception of effort. However, caffeine is a weak stimulant and has not been found to acutely increase muscle strength or to have a significant effect on body-fat content.

NUTRIENT ACTIVATORS THAT REQUIRE ADDITIONAL RESEARCH

There are many sports supplements on the market that contain nutrients that may or may not work as they are purported to. The ones included in this section are those which are supported by some science but which require additional studies to determine whether they are of any value. Among the popular nutrients that are in this category are CLA, HMB, L-carnitine, ribose, and pyruvate.

Conjugated Linoleic Acid (CLA)

Conjugated linoleic acid (CLA) is an omega-6 fatty acid found naturally in various foods that affects carbohydrate, protein, and fat metabolism and exhibits antioxidant properties. CLA has also been heavily marketed to strength athletes as a supplement that may help lessen protein catabolism, decrease body fat, and promote greater gains in strength and muscle mass during training. Some research has shown that supplemental CLA can reduce body-fat content. However, this effect has been shown only in laboratory mice that received massive quantities of CLA, which humans could never practically match pound for pound. Furthermore, results of research studies on the effects of CLA in combination with resistance training on muscle mass and strength gains have been negative. Therefore, while dietary CLA is an important nutrient, it is probably not a worthwhile supplement for reducing body fat or increasing muscle mass and strength.

Beta-hydroxy-beta-methylbutyrate (HMB)

Beta-hydroxy-beta-methylbutyrate (HMB) is a compound that is found naturally in various foods and produced in the body from proteins that contain the amino acid leucine. There is some evidence that HMB reduces muscle breakdown following exercise. Many strength and speed athletes use HMB supplements in the belief that HMB reduces recovery time and allows them to exercise more intensely, resulting in greater gains in muscle size and strength.

HMB has been widely studied. In studies by Nissen and colleagues, it was found that daily supplementation of HMB along with resistance training could increase muscle mass, reduce body fat, and increase strength in a dose-dependent manner. More recent studies, however, suggest that HMB supplementation has no effect on strength and muscle gains. So the case for HMB is still open. Fortunately, there are no reports of negative side effects associated with HMB supplements—except for the cost of buying them.

L-Carnitine

A natural compound with both vitamin-like and amino acid–like properties, L-carnitine is supplied in the diet by meats and is also manufactured in the liver and kidneys. Its primary function in the body is to transport fatty acids across the mitochondrial membrane so that they can be metabolized. L-carnitine is used medicinally in the treatment of conditions such as Alzheimer's disease and is also a popular weight-loss supplement. Some endurance athletes use it in the belief that it can increase the body's fat-burning efficiency during exercise.

However, studies have repeatedly shown that L-carnitine supplementation has no effect on fat utilization either at rest or during exercise and no effect on endurance performance. While L-carnitine is essential for fat utilization during exercise, it appears that athletes get as much as they need in the diet and that supplementation offers no additional benefit.

Ribose

Ribose is a sugar that the body produces through glucose metabolism and is in turn used in the structure of ATP. Therefore, it plays an important role in muscle energy production. Many strength athletes use ribose supplements in the belief that these supplements accelerate muscle recovery by increasing the rate of ATP synthesis after workouts.

However, studies have demonstrated unequivocally that ribose does not have this effect. For example, in a double-blind, randomized, placebo-controlled Belgian study, subjects performed an intensive regimen of lower-body strength exercises over a six-day period. Subjects who took a ribose supplement neither replenished ATP stores faster than subjects receiving a placebo nor outperformed them in the strength tests.

Pyruvate

Pyruvate is a compound that plays an important role in carbohydrate metabolism. Many athletes take pyruvate supplements as an ergogenic aid, but a recent review by Juhn at the University of Washington Medical School concludes that it has no ergogenic benefit during exercise. Some early research on rats suggested that pyruvate supplementation would promote fat loss by increasing resting metabolic rate and fat oxidation. However, more recent studies, including one by Stone and colleagues at Appalachian State University, have shown that pyruvate supplementation does not improve body composition in athletes. Nevertheless, many companies continue to market calcium pyruvate (the most popular supplement form of pyruvate).

SUMMARY

In order to have maximum effectiveness, nutrients must have the opportunity to act synergistically with other nutrients that serve as activators with respect to specific functions. In the Nutrient Timing System, the two most important activators are carbohydrate and protein (as well as certain amino acids found in proteins). Consuming individual amino acids and proteins during the Energy Phase enhances the ergogenic effects of carbohydrate consumed at the same time. Consuming carbohydrate during the anabolic phase amplifies the anabolic effects of proteins and individual amino acids. And consuming amino acids and protein during the anabolic phase also enhances glycogen replenishment.

While some nutritional supplements, such as creatine, have been proven to be beneficial to strength athletes, many others need additional substantiation. Before taking any supplement, you should look at the studies first to determine whether the claims are supported and, most important, whether the supplement is safe.

KEY TAKEAWAYS

- The Nutrient Timing System relies on making use of nutrient activation—the ability of certain nutrients to help other nutrients perform their jobs more effectively.

- The most important nutrient activators in Nutrient Timing are the mutual activators protein and carbohydrate, which influence each other's actions through insulin.

- Carbohydrate boosts protein synthesis and reduces protein degradation. Protein boosts glycogen synthesis and glucose metabolism (for more energy during workouts).

- Other anabolic nutrient activators include BCAAs, creatine, and caffeine.

The Right Macronutrients

y now it should be clear how important the timing of nutrient intake is in the effort to build muscle mass and strength. However, we don't want to give you the impression that the actual types of nutrients you consume are any less important than you thought they were. To get the full benefits of Nutrient Timing, you need to consume the *right* ingredients at the *right* time.

In this chapter, we discuss the macronutrients—protein, carbohydrate, and fat—as well as water. In Chapter 11, we turn our attention to the micronutrients: vitamins, minerals, and phytochemicals.

NOT ALL PROTEINS ARE CREATED EQUAL

Protein is the most talked-about nutrient in sports nutrition. What type of protein is best? How much protein do we need? These issues are hashed and rehashed in the popular media. Protein deserves such attention because of its many essential roles within the body. In fact, the word *protein* is derived from the Greek word meaning "of prime importance."

The protein content of skeletal muscle represents about 65 percent of the body's total protein, and it can be increased dramatically by resistance training. But protein is the basic structural material of all tissue cells, not just muscle cells. In addition, proteins—in the form of enzymes, antibodies, hormones, neurotransmitters, nutrient transporters, and cell membrane receptors—control every biochemical reaction that occurs within the body.

Proteins are generally long molecules composed of amino acid units. Of the twenty amino acids, nine are considered essential because your body cannot synthesize them; they must be consumed in your diet. (See "The Essential Amino Acids" on page 124.) The nonessential amino acids can be synthesized from one another.

The Essential Amino Acids

Histidine	Lysine	Threonine
Isoleucine	Methionine and/or cysteine	Tryptophan
Leucine	Phenylalanine and/or tyrosine	Valine

Proteins range in size from two or three amino acids (called peptides) to thousands. Although many of the foods we consume contain protein, the body does not use these proteins intact. Instead, dietary protein is broken down into amino acids, which are absorbed into the blood and transported to specific cells. There they are reassembled into the new proteins needed by those specific cells.

The average sedentary adult needs to consume 0.4–0.5 grams of protein per pound of body weight per day to maintain existing muscle mass. Most nutritionists recognize today that athletes in general, and strength athletes especially, require more protein than this. They frequently suggest intake levels of 0.6–0.7 grams per pound of body weight per day for muscle mass gains.

However, as shown in Chapter 6, additional gains can be achieved with even higher levels of protein consumption. Table 10.1 shows suggested protein intake levels for sedentary adults, active adults, and strength athletes.

TABLE 10.1. Protein Requirements for Three Different Levels of Activity

Description	Daily Protein Consumption (g/lb of body weight per day)
Sedentary	0.4–0.5
Active	0.6–0.7
Strength athletes	0.9–1.2

Protein-rich foods include beef, poultry, dairy products, fish, and many nuts and beans. Unfortunately, some of the best sources of protein are high in saturated fat. It's best to limit the proportion of protein you consume from foods that are high in saturated fats and cholesterol, including many cuts of meat and whole-milk dairy products.

Protein Powders

Protein supplements and meal-replacement products containing protein became popular among strength athletes in the early 1990s, and they maintain their popularity today. These products typically contain whey, casein, and/or soy.

There are four commonly used scientific measurements of protein quality:

1. **Protein efficiency ratio (PER)** is a measurement of the growth of animals consuming a fixed amount of dietary protein of a single type. It is considered less applicable to humans.

2. **The biological value** of a protein is a measurement of the amount of that protein that is retained from the total absorbed quantity for maintenance and growth.

3. **Net protein utilization** measures the amount of amino acids supplied by a given protein source that are used to synthesize new proteins in the body.

4. **Chemical score** is a measurement of the concentration of the nine essential amino acids in a protein source.

Table 10.2 uses all four indices to compare the three popular protein powder types to the standard protein quality reference food—the egg.

	TABLE 10.2. Comparison of Three Popular Protein Powder Types and Egg Protein			
Protein	**Protein Efficiency Ratio (PER)**	**Biological Value**	**Net Protein Utilization**	**Chemical Score**
Whey	3.0	104	92	>100
Casein	2.5	71	76	82
Soy	3.9	100	94	>100
Egg	2.2	74	61	69

WHEY PROTEIN

Whey protein is one of two protein types found in milk; the other is casein. These two dairy proteins are separated from each other in the standard cheese-making process. Whey used to be considered a useless byproduct of this process and was therefore discarded. However, when it was discovered that whey is actually a very high-quality protein, methods of distilling it into a powder containing little or no fat and lactose (milk sugar) were developed, and whey powder has since been used in a wide variety of protein supplements.

Whey protein is a complete protein that contains all nine essential amino acids. As shown in Table 10.2, whey protein compares favorably to other proteins by the four common measures of protein quality.

The concentration of branched-chain amino acids (BCAAs) is higher in whey protein (about 25 percent) than in any other protein source. The three BCAAs—leucine, isoleucine, and valine—are unique in that they can be taken up directly by skeletal muscle instead of having to be metabolized first by the liver. Because BCAAs are faster acting than other amino acids, they are able to serve as a fairly efficient muscle energy source during exercise and as a ready source of raw materials for muscle protein synthesis after exercise. Whey protein is also considered a fast-acting protein because it empties from the stomach and is absorbed into the bloodstream from the intestine faster than other proteins. Whey protein is particularly suited for use during the Energy and Anabolic Phases of NTS.

Whey protein is also rich in the precursors for glutathione. Glutathione is a peptide consisting of three amino acids: gamma-glutamic acid, cysteine, and glycine. Glutathione plays an important role in neutralizing free radicals and also serves as a potent detoxifier in the body. Whey protein has been shown to increase glutathione production.

Whey protein comes in a number of forms, including:

- **Whey protein hydrolysate.** A hydrolysate is a protein that has been broken down into its constituent amino acids. Hydrolysates are expensive and have a bitter taste.

- **Whey protein isolate.** A pure form of whey protein that has had almost all its lactose removed. This product may be useful for individuals who are lactose intolerant.

- **Whey protein concentrate.** The most common form of whey protein. It is inexpensive and can be incorporated into many types of products. In the past one of the drawbacks of whey protein concentrate was that it contained a high level of lactose. However, there are now commercially available formulas that are almost lactose free (less than 1 percent).

Vegetarian Muscle Building—An Oxymoron

John M. Berardi, C.S.C.S.

It's no secret that eating more protein throughout the day is beneficial to the strength athlete. But as protein researcher Peter Lemon says, "We don't eat protein, we eat food." Therefore, it's important to discuss which foods can best assist our muscle-building efforts.

We all know that meat is one of the highest-quality (and tastiest) protein choices, rich in vitamins and minerals. Yet some would have us believe that those tasty meats will clog up our arteries. So we're faced with a dilemma of Shakespearian proportions: To eat meat or not to eat meat. That is the question that plagues much of modern society, including weightlifters, bodybuilders, and other types of athletes. Although much of this debate is fought on subjective and emotional grounds, two things are becoming objectively clear. First, lean meats have not been found to clog up our arteries with saturated fat. Second, lean meat consumption may offer advantages when it comes to muscle building.

Dr. Wayne W. Campbell, a nutrition, exercise, and metabolism researcher from the University of Arkansas, has consistently shown that lacto-ovo-vegetarian eating (dairy and eggs are allowed) can interfere with the positive body composition changes seen in meat-eating older weight trainers. In his studies, subjects were given 0.8–1.6 grams of protein per kilogram of body weight per day. Regardless of the protein intake, vegetarians did not improve to the same degree that meat-eating trainees did. In one particular study, the meat-eating group consumed a diet containing the following protein breakdown: 17 percent dairy, 4 percent egg, 16 percent beef, 4 percent poultry, 15 percent pork, 3 percent fish, and 37 percent "other." The lacto-ovo-vegetarian group consumed a diet containing 32 percent dairy, 3 percent egg, 0 percent beef, 0 percent poultry, 0 percent pork, 0 percent fish, and 65 percent "other."

After twelve weeks of training, the meat-eating group lost about 2.9 pounds of fat while gaining about 3.7 pounds of lean mass. However, the vegetarian group gained about 0.2 pound of fat and lost about 2.4 pounds of lean mass.

The balance of Campbell's work seems to indicate that eating a varied diet that contains meat protein can lead to increased muscle mass and fat loss in conjunction with a resistance-training program. Since vegetarian proteins (besides egg and dairy) are deficient in certain essential amino acids, even with a total calculated protein intake that seems adequate, vegetarians may be limiting their muscle-building potential.

CASEIN

Casein is the other protein distilled through cheese production. It is significantly different from whey protein, as shown in Table 10.2. Although casein does not score as well as whey protein on some of the important indices, it is still an excellent source of glutamine—a crucial amino acid for strength athletes.

Two disadvantages of casein are that it has lower concentrations of BCAAs than whey and is more likely to cause gastrointestinal problems in those who are lactose sensitive or lactose intolerant.

Casein digests more slowly than whey. Although this is a disadvantage in both the Energy and Anabolic Phases, it is an advantage during the longer Growth Phase since casein is able to sustain muscle protein synthesis for a longer period. Many strength athletes take a casein supplement before going to bed to minimize protein loss during the long overnight fast.

SOY PROTEIN

Soy protein was the first powdered protein supplement to hit the market. In fact, it was originally discovered back in 1904 by George Washington Carver. Soy protein is rich in BCAAs but contains only a small amount of the essential amino acid methionine. Most forms of soy protein are highly digestible and therefore fast acting, but soy protein is generally considered a slightly lower-quality protein than whey or casein.

However, soy protein isolates fortified with methionine are now available and are of comparable quality to whey and casein. And one advantage of a soy protein isolate over whey and casein is that it contains no lactose, so those who cannot or do not consume dairy-based products can use it.

Many strength athletes avoid soy protein because it contains isoflavones (plant hormones), which have been shown to have an estrogenic effect in the body. In other words, they mimic the actions of the female sex hormone estrogen in certain tissues of the body. But this does not automatically mean that isoflavones reduce testosterone levels and inhibit muscle hypertrophy, as many have assumed. In fact, there is no evidence whatsoever that this is the case.

CARBOHYDRATES

The primary function of carbohydrates is to serve as an energy fuel for the body. As their name suggests, carbohydrates are carbon- and water-based molecules ranging in size from the very small to the very large and are abundant in most plant foods, especially fruits and grains. There are many different types of carbohydrates, ranging from simple sugars such as glucose and fructose to long polysaccharides, which may contain 300–26,000 simple sugars linked together. Regardless of the size of the carbohydrate found in food, once it has been consumed it is broken down in the stomach and intestines to the smallest unit, which is usually glucose.

Glucose is transported into the muscles and other tissues, where it is broken down further to generate energy. When glucose is not needed immediately for energy, it is stored in the muscle and liver in long chains called glycogen. The body's capacity for storing glycogen is limited. Once glycogen stores in the muscle and liver are replenished, excess glucose can be converted into fat. It is the conversion of glucose into fat that has given rise to the belief that carbohydrate is bad. Even many strength athletes strive to reduce their carbohydrate intake levels as much as possible. Extreme carbohydrate restriction is counterproductive and potentially even dangerous for athletes. Since muscle and liver glycogen stores are limited, a low-carbohydrate diet will not provide you with enough energy to perform a hard workout. In addition, since carbohydrate (as well as glutamine) provides the essential fuel for the immune system, a low-carbohydrate diet may make you more susceptible to colds and infection.

Simple and Complex Carbohydrates

Carbohydrates are divided into two basic categories: simple and complex. Simple carbohydrates contain just one or two molecules of sugars and have a sweet taste. Examples of simple carbohydrates are fructose and sucrose. Most fruits are rich in simple sugars, as are sweets and other processed foods that contain refined sugars (for instance, many breakfast cereals). Complex carbohydrates may contain hundreds or even thousands of sugars linked to form a single molecule and have a milder taste. There are two major forms of complex carbohydrates: starches and fibers. Starches are digested more slowly than simple sugars and therefore provide less energy in the short term, but more in the long term. Some foods that contain significant amounts of starch include potatoes, wheat, rice, and other grains.

There are two types of dietary fiber: soluble and insoluble. Neither is digestible, but both are essential to good health. Soluble fibers have the form of gums or pastes and dissolve in water. They have been shown to be extremely valuable in helping to lower blood cholesterol. Soluble fibers bind bile acids and remove them from the body. Bile acids are needed to make cholesterol. In the absence of bile acids, therefore, cholesterol levels are lowered.

Insoluble fiber, or cellulose, is the constituent that gives structure to plants. Cellulose provides a number of important benefits, including absorbing and removing toxins and contributing to healthy functioning of the digestive tract. Examples of fiber-rich foods are whole grains, green leafy vegetables, and beans.

The daily recommended fiber intake is 25–30 grams. The average American gets only 10 grams of fiber a day, however, so chances are you need to make some dietary modifications to increase your fiber consumption.

Glycemic Index

The glycemic index is a method of categorizing foods by their effect on blood glucose levels. A food with a low-glycemic index produces a mild, sustained increase in glucose. A food with a high-glycemic index, on the other hand, produces a larger, more transient glucose spike. At one time, conventional wisdom held that foods containing predominantly simple sugars had a high-glycemic index, while those containing predominantly complex carbohydrates had a low-glycemic index. We now know that there are many exceptions to this rule. Generally whole grains have a lower glycemic index than refined grains, high-fiber foods have a lower glycemic index than low-fiber foods, and foods containing high amounts of protein and/or fat have a lower glycemic index than foods with small amounts of protein and fat.

The general public perception is that high-glycemic carbohydrates are a bad nutritional choice because they cause insulin spikes and subsequent blood sugar crashes. This results in greater fatigue and can also trigger hunger and overeating. However, their powerful effect on insulin also makes high-glycemic sugars valuable during and immediately after exercise. They not only provide energy, but also, through their action on insulin, help reduce cortisol levels and turn on the cells' anabolic machinery. Still, as we have seen, they provide these benefits best when combined in the proper ratio with protein.

Another often-overlooked benefit of carbohydrates during extended exercise is that they help in the metabolism of fat. The muscle cell has a

Overtraining and Nutrition

John M. Berardi, C.S.C.S.

You know the feeling. You begin a new training phase pumped up and raring to go. Then, at about week six, "it" happens. First, you start feeling a little bit drained. Next, you start feeling a specific brand of muscular soreness that you haven't felt before. Finally, your motivation to get to the gym takes a dramatic downturn. While you try your best to fight through the apathy, the soreness, and the generalized fatigue, this phenomenon, known as overreaching, is stronger than you. At this point, while you've fought nobly, it's time to take a few days off: If you try to keep fighting through it, you'll slip into a much more dangerous condition known as overtraining. That's right: No matter how tough you are (physically or mentally), in the end overtraining always wins out.

According to Wilmore and Costill (1988), "No single physiological measurement has proven 100 percent effective [to diagnose overtraining]. Since performance is the most dramatic indicator of overtraining, it is not surprising to find that overtraining has a dramatic effect on the energy demands for a standard, submaximal exercise bout. When runners show symptoms of overtraining, their heart rates and oxygen consumption during the runs are significantly higher." What does this mean to you? Well, it means that there's no way to predict the arrival of overreaching or overtraining. You simply start to feel run down and, if you don't take some time off—wham—you're overtrained.

Why worry about overtraining? For starters, it leads to decreases in performance and can, if you try to train through it, result in long periods of poor performance, illness, or even injury. According to Fry and colleagues, "Overtrained subjects reported an inability to resume their normal resistance training loads for up to 8 weeks after this study, thus requiring a long-term regeneration period." This means that if you allow yourself to develop full-blown overtraining, it may be months before you'll be able to train hard again.

While little is known about preventing performance decline and overtraining, a few things are clear. First, while short periods of overreaching can be beneficial to strength and muscle gain, you must not let this overreaching go unchecked. After one week of overreaching, either decrease training volume and intensity or take a few days off.

Second, nutrition may play an important role in preventing performance decrements and overtraining. Here are some nutritional strategies for intensive training periods:

1. Consume more total calories. Overreaching and overtraining increase the metabolic cost of exercise and recovery. To prevent immune compromise, weight losses, and decreases in performance, you must eat more food.

2. Eat more carbohydrates. Some symptoms of overreaching may be caused by progressive decreases in liver muscle glycogen concentrations (even in strength athletes). Eating more carbohydrates, especially when muscle glycogen resynthesis is most efficient (during the postworkout period), will ensure adequate liver and muscle carbohydrate stores.

3. Eat more dietary fat. While low-fat diets were all the rage in the 1980s and 1990s, new research has demonstrated that certain types of dietary fat can offer protection against heart disease, free-radical damage, and cancer, and can increase metabolic rate and fat burning, muscle mass, and the production of hormones such as testosterone. During overtraining, testosterone concentrations in the blood tend to decrease. Increasing the amount of fat in your diet may help prevent some of this decline.

4. Ingest a good postexercise carbohydrate/protein drink. After exercise, the body is primed for muscle glycogen resynthesis and the repair of muscle damage. A carbohydrate/protein drink based on the principles of the Nutrient Timing System can improve muscle glycogen recovery and muscle protein status. Furthermore, during overtraining, cortisol concentrations in the blood may increase. Postexercise nutrition containing carbohydrates and protein may prevent some of this rise in cortisol.

metabolic priority system when it comes to which nutrients it uses for energy. For short exercise bouts such as sets of resistance exercise, carbohydrate is the primary nutrient used. During extended exercise the muscles rely increasingly on fat stores. But carbohydrate is still required to drive the use of fat for energy. In this sense, "fats burn in a carbohydrate flame." After forty-five minutes of exercise, protein—primarily BCAAs—can provide up to 15 percent of a muscle's total energy needs.

Table 10.3 details the glycemic index ratings of common foods. An important principle of the NTS is selective consumption of high-glycemic sugars before, during and after your workout.

TABLE 10.3. Glycemic Index Ratings of Some Common Foods		
High GI	**Moderate GI**	**Low GI**
Cornflakes	Bran muffin	Apple
Honey	Oatmeal	Low-fat milk
Baked potato	Spaghetti (plain)	Pear
Sports drink	Apple juice	Banana
Bagel	White rice	Whole milk
White bread	Brown rice	Barley
Watermelon	Strawberries	Grapefruit
Cheerios	Peas	Peach
Wheat bread	Kidney beans	Dried apricots

FATS

It is ironic that sugar is considered the "bad" macronutrient and fat is considered the "unhealthy" one. In fact, both nutrients are essential for a healthy diet. Problems arise when excesses are consumed.

Fats serve many functions in the body. They are the most energy-dense macronutrient, and they provide many of the body's tissues and organs (including the heart) with most of their energy. Cell membranes are partly composed of a specific type of fat called phospholipids. Fats are critical for the transmission of nerve signals that generate muscle contractions, they serve as a transporter for vitamins A, D, E, and K, and they provide cushioning for the protection of vital organs and insulation from the thermal stress of cold environments. Finally, because fat empties more slowly from the stomach, it helps delay the onset of hunger pangs. This is one reason why diets containing moderate amounts of fat tend to be more successful than low-fat diets.

Fat is an ideal fuel for muscle cells because per gram it contains almost twice the energy of glucose, it weighs less per volume, and it is easily transported and stored. In healthy males, fat constitutes approximately 15 percent of body mass; in healthy females, about 25 percent.

All fats are composed of fatty acids, which are usually linked in three-unit molecules called triglycerides. There are three major types of fatty acids—saturated, polyunsaturated, and monounsaturated—distinguished by their molecular bonds and the number of hydrogen atoms they contain. Saturated fats are typically solid at room temperature and are found in the greatest abundance in meats and dairy foods. Monounsaturated fats are liquid at room temperature and are most concentrated in oils such as olive, peanut, and canola. Polyunsaturated fats are also most abundant in certain plant oils—particularly corn and soybean oils—as well as in seeds, whole grains, and fatty types of fish (such as salmon and tuna).

Polyunsaturated fats are also known as essential fatty acids because our bodies need them but cannot make them from other nutrients. Omega-3 fatty acid is an essential fatty acid that is rare in the typical American diet; in fact, most Americans don't get enough of it. It is believed that adequate intake of omega-3 fatty acids is needed to reduce postworkout muscle inflammation and accelerate repair. Inadequate omega-3 fatty acid intake, coupled with much higher levels of omega-6 fatty acid intake, is associated with a host of degenerative diseases including heart disease, autoimmune diseases, and diabetes. Perhaps the most practical way to ensure that you get enough omega-3 fatty acids, and to put your intake of omega-6 and omega-3 fatty acids in the proper balance (a ratio of 3:1 or less), is to take a daily flaxseed oil supplement.

Trans-fatty acids (or simply trans fats) are a form of saturated fat that is unhealthy in any amount. Trans fats are a product of hydrogenation, a chemical process by which hydrogen is added to unsaturated fatty acids in order to create a solid, spreadable fat with increased shelf life. They are found in many packaged, processed baked goods and snack foods. Research shows that trans fats clog arteries, interfere with insulin function and liver detoxification, and increase the risk of heart attack and stroke.

For exercise performance, muscle growth, and general health, it is also important to limit your intake of saturated fats to no more than about 30 percent of your total fat intake. Saturated fat is not inherently bad, as many people believe. On the contrary, it is as useful as any other fat. However, *excessive* saturated fat consumption increases levels of LDL cholesterol in the blood, which in turn can lead to hypertension, stroke, heart attack, and other health problems.

In total, fat should account for 30 to 35 percent of the calories in your daily diet. There is most certainly such a thing as too little fat. When total fat intake dips below 20 percent of total calories, other health problems, such as fatigue and a weakened immune system, can result.

WATER

Water is not technically a macronutrient, but it is much like the macronutrients protein, carbohydrate, and fat in that it's an essential nutrient that we need in large amounts. In fact, we require much more water on a volume basis than we do protein, carbohydrate, and fat combined. The average human body is more than 60 percent water. Adequate water intake is necessary for proper digestion, elimination of wastes, joint lubrication, and other essential functions. Poor hydration also compromises an athlete's performance by keeping blood volume below its optimal level. Without adequate water intake, the Nutrient Timing System will not be as effective.

Daily water intake needs are highly individual. They depend on factors that include body weight, the weather, other dietary considerations such as intake of alcohol (which increases water needs), and activity level (or training volume). The average person requires roughly 1 ounce of water per kilogram of body weight on a daily basis. Athletes generally need a little more. There's no precise way to determine exactly how much water you need. It's best if athletes simply carry a water bottle at all times and sip from it at regular intervals throughout the day. Note that most foods contain water, so it's not necessary to consume a full ounce of plain water per kilogram of body weight per day.

SUMMARY

You can't build a great physique with poor nutrition. Your health and performance will pay a price for every "empty calorie" you consume, and will benefit from every improvement you make in the quality of the nutrition you take in each day.

The cornerstone of good nutrition is an appropriate balance of 19 to 26 percent proteins, 41 to 48 percent carbohydrates, and 33 percent fats, from quality sources. If you get the right proportions and the right total amount of macronutrient calories from mainly natural whole-food sources, supplementing with proven-effective supplements such as the protein powders discussed in this chapter, you're halfway to achieving an optimal nutrition regimen for muscle growth. The rest is timing.

KEY TAKEAWAYS

- To promote maximum muscle growth, you need to maintain a high-protein diet of at least 2.0 grams per kilogram of body weight per day.

- Emphasize high-quality proteins such as whey protein over lower quality proteins such as plant-food proteins.

- Try to consume mostly low- and moderate-glycemic carbohydrates during the Growth Phase for consistent energy, less hunger, and greater nutrient density.

- Limit the amount of saturated and trans fats (which clog arteries) in your diet and be sure to get enough omega-3 fatty acids, which reduce postworkout inflammation and accelerate tissue repair.

- Nutrition strategies such as increasing healthy-fat intake can (alongside rest, of course) help you overcome overtraining.

The Right Micronutrients

Micronutrients are organic compounds called vitamins and inorganic minerals that the body requires in very small amounts. Vitamins and minerals are considered essential because they cannot be synthesized in the body; they must be consumed in food. In this chapter, we discuss the functions of several vitamins and minerals that are particularly important to strength athletes and give a nod to those amazing plant nutrients, the phytochemicals.

VITAMINS

There are thirteen essential vitamins. All act as catalysts, speeding up the various chemical reactions that our lives depend on. Without vitamins to catalyze these reactions, they could not take place quickly enough to support life.

The body cannot synthesize vitamins, so they must be consumed consistently in adequate amounts in foods and supplements. There are two basic categories of vitamins: water soluble and fat soluble. The body can store the fat-soluble vitamins A, D, E, and K in small amounts within fat tissues, but it cannot store the water-soluble vitamins (B complex and C), so it's especially important to consume these daily.

The B-vitamin complex and vitamins C, D, and E are especially important for strength athletes.

B-Vitamin Complex

The eight vitamins that make up the B-vitamin complex are thiamine (B_1), riboflavin (B_2), niacin (B_3), pyridoxine (B_6), folate (B_9), cyanocobalamin (B_{12}), pantothenic acid (B_5), and biotin. As a group, these nutrients are vital coenzymes that aid in releasing energy from carbohydrates, fats, and proteins. Vitamin B_6 also assists in building proteins from amino acids. Vitamin B_{12} and folate play important roles in cellular reproduction and red blood cell synthesis.

Most of the B vitamins in the diet come attached to proteins in the foods we eat. A diet that contains high amounts of protein-rich foods such as meats, nuts, and beans provides plenty of B vitamins. Folate is found in the greatest abundance in green leafy vegetables and is the only member of the B-vitamin complex in which many people are deficient. You can ensure adequate folate intake by adding more green leafy vegetables to your diet and by taking a daily multivitamin with folate. See Table 11.1 for recommended daily intake amounts of each of the B vitamins.

Vitamin C

Vitamin C is perhaps the most multitasking nutrient in humans. It is the only vitamin that is present in every cell of the body. On a structural level, it is a major ingredient of collagen, a protein that connects cells to form tissues. Vitamin C is also a potent antioxidant that neutralizes free-radical molecules before they can damage lipid cells. Free-radical damage is a major factor in aging and in the development of many degenerative diseases such as cancer.

Vitamin C helps replenish supplies of vitamin E, another important antioxidant. It also assists iron absorption and fat metabolism. Also, new evidence suggests that vitamin C supplementation may blunt the release of the catabolic hormone cortisol during especially hard workouts. In one study, ultramarathon runners who took 1,000 milligrams of supplemental vitamin C per day for the seven days preceding a ninety-kilometer run exhibited 30 percent lower cortisol levels immediately after the race and therefore very likely experienced much less muscle tissue breakdown.

Vitamin C also protects the body against viral infections, which athletes in heavy training are at greater risk of. One study showed that daily supplementation of 600 mg of ascorbic acid (vitamin C) significantly reduced the incidence of upper respiratory infections in individuals who participated in a marathon. In another study by Peters and colleagues, an antioxidant combination consisting of vitamin C, vitamin E, and beta-carotene decreased upper respiratory infections by almost 40 percent. Similar results have been seen by other investigators.

Because exercise greatly increases the body's use of oxygen, which is a free radical, athletes use more vitamin C to neutralize free radicals than sedentary people and therefore require more vitamin C in their diet. An intake of 800–2,000 milligrams a day is recommended for active adults. Exceeding this dosage may result in a number of side effects, including diarrhea and joint pain. Good sources of vitamin C include many fruits (such as oranges, grapefruits, and strawberries) and vegetables (such as tomatoes, broccoli, green and red bell peppers, and leafy greens).

Vitamin D

The function of vitamin D is to maintain normal blood levels of calcium and phosphorus. Vitamin D facilitates the absorption of calcium, which is essential to the formation and maintenance of strong, healthy bones. It works in concert with a number of other vitamins, minerals, and hormones to keep the bones mineral-dense. Weightlifters need especially strong bones due to the extreme forces they are routinely subjected to in the gym.

Vitamin D is actually very rare in natural foods. The only foods that contain vitamin D in high amounts are fatty fish and fish oil. Eggs and beef contain small amounts. Most of the vitamin D in the typical American diet is obtained through vitamin-D-fortified milk and breakfast cereals. Interestingly, sun exposure results in vitamin D synthesis in the body, so those who get plenty of sun require less vitamin D in the diet. Athletes need 400–1,000 IU (international units; 1 IU = 0.45 mg) per day.

Vitamin E

Vitamin E is a fat-soluble vitamin that comes in eight forms, the most prevalent and useful of which is alpha-tocopherol. Vitamin E is a powerful antioxidant. It protects cells, including muscle cells, from destruction at the hands of free radicals by helping maintain cell membrane integrity. This protection accelerates postworkout recovery in three ways: It limits the loss of muscle proteins, lessens postworkout inflammation, and reduces postworkout muscle soreness.

A number of good studies have demonstrated the recovery-aiding benefits of vitamin E in those who engage in strenuous exercise. In one recent study, thirty-two healthy men were randomly assigned to take a daily 1,000 IU vitamin E supplement or a placebo for twelve weeks and ran downhill (which causes more muscle damage than flat running because it puts more eccentric stress on the muscles) for forty-five minutes at 75 percent VO_2 max (maximum rate of oxygen consumption), once before and once following supplementation. Blood samples were obtained before and immediately postexercise, and at six, twenty-four, and seventy-two hours postexercise to assess antioxidant status, muscle damage, lipid peroxidation, and DNA damage. The researchers found that vitamin E supplementation had a statistically significant beneficial effect on exercise-induced muscle damage.

Vitamin E may also have a beneficial effect on the immune system. Several studies have shown that vitamin E supplementation improves a number of immune system elements. Whether it does so directly or by counteracting the immunosuppressive effects of cortisol is not known.

Interestingly, vitamin E seems to be more effective as a recovery aid when used in combination with vitamin C. These two antioxidants work synergistically, in complementary ways, as mutual activators. Recommended daily intake of vitamin E for strength athletes is 200–1,000 IU. Good sources of vitamin E include green leafy vegetables, legumes, nuts, seeds, and whole grains.

Table 11.1. The Essential Vitamins

Vitamin	RDI* for Adult Athletes
Vitamin A	5,000–25,000 IU
Vitamin B_1 (thiamine)	30–200 mg
Vitamin B_2 (riboflavin)	30–200 mg
Vitamin B_3 (niacin)	20–100 mg
Vitamin B_5 (pantothenic acid)	25–200 mg
Vitamin B_6 (pyridoxine)	20–100 mg
Vitamin B_{12} (cobalamin)	12–200 mcg**
Biotin	125–250 mcg**
Folate (folic acid, vitamin B_9)	400–1,000 mcg**
Vitamin C	800–2,000 mg
Vitamin D	400–1,000 IU
Vitamin E	200–1,000 IU
Vitamin K	80–180 mcg**

*Recommended Daily Intake   **Micrograms; 1 mcg = 0.001 mg.

MINERALS

Minerals are inorganic nutrients that are absorbed into plants from the earth's surface and then make their way into our bodies when we eat those plants or eat animals that have eaten plants. The most important minerals for muscle building are calcium, iron, phosphorus, and zinc. Also of special value for all active persons are the electrolyte minerals magnesium, potassium, sodium, and chloride.

Calcium

When we think of calcium, we usually think of bones. And it's true that 99 percent of the calcium in the human body is contained in bones as calcium phosphate. However, calcium also plays critical roles in muscle action and muscle growth. Positively charged calcium ions located at neuromuscular junctions are needed to turn an electrical impulse from the brain into a chemical action that causes muscle fibers to contract and relax. Calcium ions also help regulate muscle glycogen breakdown and the oxidation of carbohydrates during exercise.

Everyone knows that dairy products are excellent sources of calcium, but so are many types of seafood (shellfish, salmon, shrimp) and vegetables (broccoli, kale, collard greens). Adults who regularly participate in strenuous exercise require 1,200–2,600 milligrams of calcium per day. But in order to be properly absorbed, calcium requires the help of other nutrient activators, especially magnesium. You need to consume approximately 1 milligram of magnesium for every 2 grams of calcium for optimal calcium absorption.

Iron

Iron is a trace mineral (that is, a mineral needed in very small amounts) that is necessary for the formation of hemoglobin, the oxygen-carrying compound found in red blood cells. Since oxygen plays a vital role in breaking down carbohydrates and fats for energy, especially during exercise, iron serves as an indirect nutrient activator for carbohydrates and fats. Fatigue is the primary symptom of iron deficiency.

Despite the low levels of iron humans require, iron deficiency is relatively common in female athletes. Women and girls tend to consume less iron in their diets than men and boys. At the same time, high levels of activity increase iron needs. Menstruation further increases iron losses. These factors put female athletes at a higher risk of anemia.

Iron-rich foods include meat, fish, eggs, dark green leafy vegetables, and certain beans, whole grains, and nuts. Men and women who work out frequently require 10–20 milligrams of iron per day.

Magnesium

Magnesium is found in all the body's cells, but is most concentrated in the bones, muscles, and soft tissues. It's a necessary element in over 300 enzyme reactions involving nerve transmission, muscle contraction, and especially energy release from ATP. Low blood magnesium levels during exercise have also been cited as causing muscle fatigue and irregular heartbeat.

Good food sources of magnesium are apples, avocados, bananas, brown rice, dairy foods, garlic, green leafy vegetables, legumes, nuts, soybeans, and whole grains. The recommended daily intake for athletes is 400–800 milligrams.

Phosphorus

Phosphorus is the second most abundant mineral in the body, after calcium. It is a constituent of the two most important sources of energy for maximum-intensity efforts—ATP and creatine phosphate. In the bones, it binds to calcium to form calcium phosphate. It also binds with lipids to form phospholipids, which make up cell membranes. In addition, phosphorus plays a role in the metabolism of carbohydrate and fat.

Good food sources of phosphorus are milk, fish, eggs, asparagus, corn, legumes, nuts, meats, poultry, salmon, and some seeds. The recommended daily intake for athletes is 800–1,600 milligrams.

Potassium

Potassium is necessary for nerve transmission, muscle contraction, and glycogen formation. It also aids in maintaining cardiovascular system function. During workouts, potassium helps calcium do its job of stimulating muscle contractions. While it is calcium that actually stimulates the contraction, it cannot do so without the aid of potassium. Excessive potassium loss can cause muscles to contract involuntarily, resulting in painful cramps that can stop you in your tracks. In addition, potassium losses can lead to heat intolerance.

Good food sources of potassium are bananas, tomatoes, oranges, potatoes, winter squash, avocados, and beans. The recommended daily intake for athletes is 2,500–4,000 mg.

Sodium and Chloride

We mention sodium and chloride together because most of the sodium and chloride we get from foods is consumed in the form of sodium chloride—better known as table salt. Both are electrolytes, meaning they are special minerals that are electrically charged. They play key roles in maintaining fluid balance and facilitating muscle contraction and relaxation. Sodium and chloride cooperate with water to help maintain the volume and balance of all the fluids outside the body's cells, such as blood.

Sodium plays a particularly important role because it helps transport nutrients into cells, so they can be used for energy production as well as tissue growth and repair. In addition, sodium functions in muscle contraction and nerve impulse transmission. Excessive loss of body sodium is known as hyponatremia, and it can be dangerous. This condition is rarely seen, however, except among ultra-endurance athletes competing in warm or hot weather.

Sources of sodium chloride are table salt, sea salt, and most processed foods (such as snack chips, processed baked goods, and frozen entrées). The recommended daily intake of sodium and chloride for athletes is 1,500–4,500 milligrams. The average American consumes 6,000 milligrams of sodium chloride daily.

Zinc

Zinc is present in every cell of the body and is a constituent of more than 300 enzymes that catalyze the chemical reactions our lives depend on. The mechanisms of zinc's actions are still poorly understood, but we do know that it plays important roles in tissue repair and maintenance and immune system function. Due to its role in tissue repair and its ability to raise testosterone levels, zinc is considered an anabolic mineral. Good sources of zinc include shellfish, beef, lamb, free-range eggs, lentils, almonds, and chicken. Daily recommended intake for athletes is 15–60 milligrams.

PHYTOCHEMICALS

Phytochemicals are plant chemicals other than macronutrients, vitamins, and minerals; they can serve as nutrients within the human body. Although they are not considered essential nutrients, phytochemicals

Table 11.2. The Essential Minerals

Mineral	RDI* for Adult Athletes
Boron	5–10 mg
Calcium	1,200–2,600 mg
Chloride	1,500–4,500 mg
Chromium	200–400 mcg**
Copper	3–6 mg
Iodine	200–400 mcg**
Iron	10–20 mg
Magnesium	400–800 mg
Manganese	15–45 mg
Molybdenum	100–300 mcg**
Phosphorus	800–1,600 mg
Potassium	2,500–4,000 mg
Selenium	100–300 mcg**
Sodium	1,500–4,500 mg
Sulfur	None established
Zinc	15–60 mg

*Recommended Daily Intake   **Micrograms; 1 mcg = 0.001 mg.

have tremendous and wide-ranging powers to improve our health and therefore should be considered essential for optimal health.

There are literally thousands of different phytochemicals, most of which have not yet been identified. Dozens have been identified, however, and their beneficial effects studied. Many phytochemicals are antioxidants. Lutein is a phytochemical found in green leafy vegetables that has been proven to prevent macular degeneration, an eye disease with an apparent link to oxidative damage. Beta-carotene protects the immune system. Capsaicin discourages tumor growth. And the list goes on.

Our reductionist nutrition mentality tempts us to turn individual phytochemicals into supplements and to take them in heavy doses; however, the evidence suggests that phytochemicals are effective only when consumed in the balance in which they are found in whole foods. This is one reason why it is important that we get the majority of our daily calories from whole foods, and particularly whole plant foods.

SUMMARY

Vitamins and minerals are not something you need to spend too much time thinking about. While they are critical not just to muscle performance but also to general health, meeting your body's vitamin and mineral needs for optimal health and fitness is easy. Simply maintain plenty of balance and variety in your diet, fill up mainly on natural, whole foods, and perhaps take a daily multivitamin and multimineral supplement for insurance, and you'll be good to go. There are no timing issues with respect to micronutrient intake beyond the general need for *daily* consumption.

KEY TAKEAWAYS

- *Maintain a balanced diet with plenty of variety to ensure you get all the vitamins and minerals your body needs daily.*

- *The antioxidant vitamins C and E are especially important for athletes due to their proven ability to reduce exercise-related free-radical damage.*

- *Iron deficiencies are not uncommon in athletes, and especially female athletes, but with monitoring it's very easy to maintain adequate iron levels in the blood.*

- *Don't forget about the phytochemicals—although not technically essential, these nutrients are powerful health boosters and are present abundantly in fruits, vegetables, and whole grains.*

- *Take a daily multivitamin and multimineral supplement for insurance.*

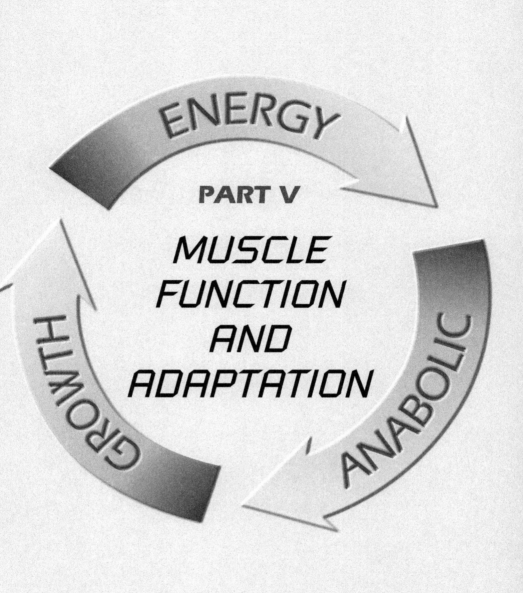

ENERGY

ANABOLIC

GROWTH

PART V

*MUSCLE
FUNCTION
AND
ADAPTATION*

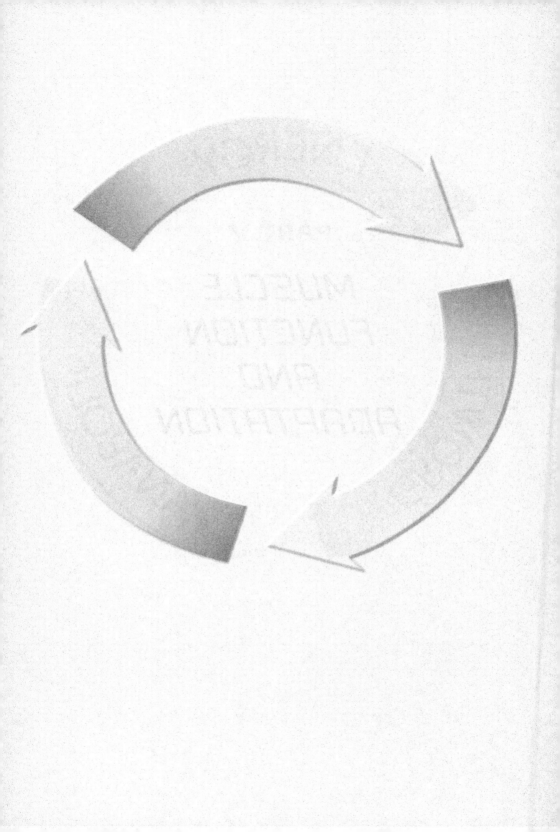

How Muscles Work and Adapt to Training

Muscles are extraordinary organs that appear to be rather simply constructed, but in reality, they are highly sophisticated and adaptable structures. Muscle makes up about 40 to 45 percent of the body weight of men and about 35 to 40 percent of the body weight of women. Of course, these percentages can be greatly increased with the proper exercise training and nutrition protocol. Improving the size, strength, and power of your muscles requires more than just hard work. It requires that the appropriate *type* of work be performed, and it also requires that you have a sound nutrition plan that allows you to get the most out of your workouts. In order to design an effective exercise program and nutrition plan to meet these goals, one must base them on a solid understanding of how muscles work and how they adapt to exercise training.

Nutrient Timing is the exercise nutrition program that best exploits our current knowledge about the way muscles function during and between workouts. The purpose of this chapter is to provide you with a foundation in this knowledge. You won't need to retain every detail in order to practice Nutrient Timing effectively, but it is important to grasp the general concepts.

MUSCLE STRUCTURE

If you were to cut through a muscle, you would see that it is made up of bundles separated by connective tissue (see Figure 12.1). These bundles, called fasciculi, are made up of individual muscle fibers, or cells. Unlike other cells of the body, muscle fibers have several nuclei, possibly because of their exceptional length. In some of the larger muscles of the body, such as the thigh muscles, muscle fibers can exceed twelve inches in length.

Muscle fibers are further subdivided into myofibrils and the myofibrils into sarcomeres. The sarcomeres are the smallest functional units of a muscle fiber and consist of the major contractile proteins myosin and actin. These proteins are long filaments arranged in a parallel formation. During contraction, the actin filament is pulled toward the center of the sarcomere by the myosin filament, causing the sarcomere to shorten. Shortening of the sarcomeres in a myofibril causes the shortening of the muscle fiber. Within a muscle, the number of muscle fibers contracting at any given time is determined by the amount of force required to overcome the resistance to movement and shorten the muscle. For example, curling 10 pounds requires fewer muscle fibers to be recruited than curling 20 pounds.

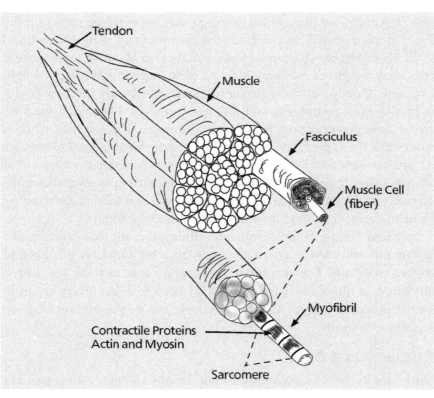

Figure 12.1. Muscle Structure
Muscle is composed of bundles of muscle fibers called fasciculi. The muscle fibers are divided into myofibrils, and myofibrils are divided into sarcomeres, the smallest functional unit of the muscle fiber. Sarcomeres consist of the major contractile proteins, myosin and actin.

MUSCLE FIBER TYPES

Not all muscle fibers are the same. Skeletal muscles contain two basic fiber types, each with its own contractile and metabolic profile. Having different types of muscle fibers allows the muscles to have a more diverse performance capability. The two types of fibers are referred to as slow-twitch (type I) and fast-twitch (type II) fibers. Compared with fast-twitch fibers, slow-twitch fibers are slow to contract and relax, but have a high number of mitochondria, allowing them a greater aerobic-energy capacity. Slow-twitch fibers are surrounded by a larger number of small blood vessels called capillaries that bring in oxygen and nutrients and carry away waste products. Conversely, fast-twitch fibers contract and relax faster than slow-twitch fibers and have a greater glycolytic capacity. They also have a greater store of the high-energy phosphates and glycogen, but have fewer mitochondria and capillaries.

Because of their contractile and metabolic characteristics, slow-twitch fibers do not fatigue as easily as fast-twitch fibers and are therefore used for high-endurance activities. Fast-twitch fibers contract rapidly and function well anaerobically, or without oxygen, for short periods of time. These fibers are responsible for strength and speed. They are recruited during high-intensity activities that demand quick bursts of energy, such as sprinting, jumping, and stop-and-go movements that occur in sports such as basketball and baseball. However, fast-twitch fibers fatigue quickly due to the buildup of lactic acid, a byproduct of anaerobic metabolism.

Everyone has both types of fibers in their muscles, but the relative amount that a person has is genetically determined and can vary widely from one person to the next. For most individuals, muscle fiber type composition is in the range of 50 percent slow-twitch and 50 percent fast-twitch fibers. However, it is possible for the proportion of fibers to be skewed toward one extreme or the other and this can greatly affect athletic potential. For example, elite marathon runners are likely to possess a high percentage of slow-twitch fibers in their muscles, whereas sprinters are likely to possess a high percentage of fast-twitch fibers in their muscles. All muscle fibers, however, can respond to athletic training by improving their ability to perform according to the way they are trained. Accordingly, training aerobically can increase the mitochondrial content and aerobic metabolic capacity of fast-twitch fibers, and training anaerobically will enhance the phosphagen system of the slow-twitch fibers.

Table 12.1 lists the physiological characteristic of muscle fiber.

TABLE 12.1. Physiological Characteristics of Muscle Fiber Types

	Fiber Types	
Physiological Characteristics	**Slow Twitch**	**Fast Twitch**
Fiber size	Small	Large
Contraction velocity	Slow	Fast
Relaxation velocity	Slow	Fast
Fatigue resistance	High	Low
Aerobic capacity	High	Low
Anaerobic capacity	Low	High
Mitochondria density	High	Low
Creatine phosphate content	Low	High
Glycogen content	Low	High
Fat content	High	Low
Capillary density	High	Low

DETERMINATION OF FORCE AND SPEED OF CONTRACTION

Force and speed of muscle contraction are governed by the type and number of muscle fibers recruited or activated, as well as by the frequency of their activation. Slow-twitch fibers are first to be recruited and then fast-twitch fibers are recruited. This allows for the systematic mobilization of muscle fibers to accommodate the specific tension, speed, and metabolic requirements of muscle contraction. In general, slow-twitch fibers are recruited during low-intensity exercise. This is followed by activation of the more powerful fast-twitch fibers as the muscle-force requirements increase. When low-intensity activity is prolonged, slow-twitch fibers are initially recruited, but as they fatigue, there is a progressive involvement of fast-twitch fibers.

The differential control of muscle fiber recruitment patterns is a major factor in determining success in various athletic activities. For example, weightlifters are capable of recruiting a high number of slow- and fast-twitch fibers together in what is referred to as a synchronous pattern. This synchronous pattern of muscle fiber recruitment aids the weightlifter in generating high amounts of force quickly. Conversely, the endurance athlete recruits muscle fibers sequentially, or asynchronously, depending heavily on the high-oxidative slow-twitch fibers. The asynchronous recruitment pattern is advantageous because it provides a recovery period for the muscle fibers during the activity.

HOW MUSCLES ADAPT

The process by which muscles adapt to exercise training is not straightforward. As any athlete is keenly aware, different training programs result in different metabolic and physiological adaptations. We only have to compare the strength athlete with the endurance athlete to see the extreme range of effects of exercise training on the body. Even with training programs of equal caloric expenditure, the endurance athlete is not going to develop a measurable amount of muscle mass, and the strength athlete is not going to have an increase in aerobic capacity. Even different weightlifting programs can bring about completely different results. In short, the adaptations to training are highly specific to the type of training that is performed. Furthermore, there is considerable individual variation in response to the same training program. This is in large part due to one's genetic potential. It can also be significantly influenced by nutritional intervention.

Let's now consider how muscles adapt and the influence that exercise can have on their development.

BASIC PRINCIPLES OF EXERCISE TRAINING

There are four basic principles of exercise training that you should understand if you are going to design a training program that meets your specific needs. Table 12.2 on page 154 provides a brief overview of these principles. You can of course copy what other athletes are doing in their training programs, but everyone responds differently. Therefore, for the best possible training benefits, your training program should be individualized.

TABLE 12.2. Basic Principles of Exercise Training

Principle	Comment
1. Specificity	Adaptations are specific to the activity, volume, and intensity of exercise.
2. Progressive overload	For adaptation to occur, the overload on a specific muscle must be greater than normally encountered.
3. Disuse	Adaptations are not permanent.
4. Individuality	Capacity to adapt is in large part determined by your genetic makeup.

Principle 1: Specificity of Exercise

The principle of exercise specificity states that the biological adaptations to training are specific to the activity and to the volume and intensity of the exercise performed. Therefore, improvements are restricted to the energy systems, muscle groups, and other biological systems stressed during training. For example, a resistance-training program that emphasizes low weight, high repetitions, and a moderate number of sets will increase muscle endurance, but will not maximize strength gains and muscle development. A program of high-weight, moderate repetitions, and a high number of sets will emphasize muscle development, but not necessarily maximize muscle-strength development.

Even the speed with which you complete the concentric (weight-raising) and eccentric (weight-lowering) phases of a lift will have an effect on muscle adaptation. In most sports, it is important that the development of muscle strength emphasize functional strength or explosive power. To best obtain this type of strength, some of your sets should be designed so that the concentric phase of the lift is performed as rapidly as possible. Strength development using a slow concentric contraction does not necessarily result in an increase in strength at faster speeds of contraction. Consequently, a shot-putter's strength-training program should incorporate sets of shoulder presses and squats in which the concentric phase of each exercise is performed in an explosive manner. Therefore, based on the principle of specificity, your training program should stress the physiological systems that are critical for optimal performance in a way that best simulates how they are to be used.

Principle 2: Progressive Overload

Overload refers to a physiological stress or level of exercise that is beyond what is customary. Progressive refers to a continued increase in the level of overload. The overload principle states that, for a training adaptation to occur, the load or stress on the system or systems of the body being trained must be greater than typically encountered. Once the system adapts to the increased stress of training, the stress is no longer atypical, and if further training adaptations are desired, the training stimulus must be increased. Consider a football player with a starting bench press of 300 pounds. After one month of training with 210 pounds (3 sets x 10 reps x 3 times per week), his 1 repetition maximum (1RM) increases to 315 pounds. If this individual continues to train the next month using the same training protocol he used the first month, he will not see any appreciable improvement in his 1RM. This is because his muscles have adapted and his training program no longer overloads his muscles. To see an additional increase in benchpress strength, he will now be required to increase his workout. Continuous improvement, therefore, requires that the level of training increase or progress as the system being trained improves.

Principle 3: Disuse

The principle of disuse can be simply defined by the saying "use it or lose it." Training adaptations are not permanent. Once you remove the stimulus for change, or the training overload, the system previously being trained will revert back to a level that will accommodate the normal daily demands placed on it. We are all aware that if one stops weightlifting, muscle atrophy will start to occur. Likewise, the muscle mitochondria of a distance runner will significantly decline if the runner stops training. However, the maintenance of a training adaptation does not require the same training overload as the original development of the adaptation. Therefore, there can be periods of time in your training program when the training overload can be lowered without significant loss of training adaptation.

Principle 4: Individuality

The capacity to adapt to exercise training is in large part genetically determined. Genetics play a major role in how fast and to what degree you will adapt to a training program. Surely you have noticed that some individuals seem only to have to look at a weight and they put on muscle, while others appear to work extremely hard with little to show for it. Because you may respond well to one type of exercise stimulus, however, does not mean that you will respond to all types of exercise stimuli. For example, someone who responds well to a weight-training program may not respond well to an endurance-training program and vice versa.

A caveat to the principle of individuality is that the further you are from your genetic potential, the easier it is to adapt to training, and the closer you are to your genetic potential, the harder it becomes to adapt. Large gains in strength are seen at the onset of a training program and adaptation is rather easy. However, after several months of training, an increase in strength can become difficult and adaptations plateau. To continue to adapt, variation must be introduced into your training program, and as you have learned, control of your nutrient intake can be of significant benefit as well.

TRAINING ADAPTATIONS

As we discussed above, the adaptations to a training program are highly specific. Before we address how the body controls muscle fiber adaptation, it is important to understand which major adaptations occur in response to different types of training. Let's look at why one exercise program increases strength while another increases muscle endurance.

Endurance Training Adaptations

After several months of endurance training, individuals are generally capable of exercising at higher workloads while maintaining sufficient energy production aerobically. They are capable of exercising for prolonged periods of time at exercise intensities that had previously resulted in early fatigue. The adaptations that result in improved aerobic power and endurance reside both in the cardiovascular system and within the skeletal muscle.

The cardiovascular system adaptations occur in the heart and blood vessels. As a result of endurance training, heart weight and volume increase. The increase in heart weight is due to an increase in wall thickness as the myocardium (heart muscle) undergoes hypertrophy (an increase in size). There is also an increase in left ventricular chamber size. The increase in left ventricular chamber size and wall thickness makes the heart a more efficient pump, and it is able to pump more blood per beat. This results in greater maximal blood flow and oxygen delivery to the working muscles during a maximal effort. Other cardiovascular adaptations include an increase in blood volume, a decrease in blood pressure, and an increase in muscle capillary density, or the number of capillaries around each muscle fiber. The increase in capillary density is important because it improves the dispersal of oxygen and nutrients into the cell and the removal of byproducts of metabolism, including carbon dioxide and lactic acid.

Endurance training also has a substantial impact on the metabolic pathways of skeletal muscle. The major adaptation is an increase in the size and number of mitochondria. This increase in mitochondria results in an increase in the lactate threshold, the workload at which blood lactic acid starts to accumulate and cause fatigue, a sparing of stored carbohydrates (glycogen), and an increased reliance on fat as a fuel source. The increased reliance on fat and the sparing of glycogen during prolonged exercise play a major role in the increase in endurance performance after training. Other metabolic adaptations include an increase in the proteins that control muscle glucose uptake and its conversion into glycogen. Because of these adaptations, endurance athletes are better able to replenish their muscle glycogen stores postexercise than untrained individuals.

Resistance Training Adaptations

The adaptations that occur with resistance training are both neurological and physiological. During the first two to three months of strength training, the major gains in strength occur because of changes in the connective tissues and nervous system. With resistance training, there is an increase in tendon, ligament, and internal connective tissue strength. The tendons of the muscle have built-in sensors that monitor muscle tension. These sensors are designed to prevent the muscle from generating more tension than the connective tissue can safely tolerate. If the muscle is developing too much tension these sensors are activated and reduce nerve stimulation to the muscle. This reduces muscle force and prevents injury to the connective tissue. As the connective tissues become stronger, activation of these sensors requires greater muscle tension (meaning that more weight can be lifted). There is also an increase in the coordination of muscle fiber recruitment, which results in better synchronization of muscle fiber contraction and force development. In other words, the more muscle fibers can be activated at the same time, the more force can be generated by the muscle during a maximal effort.

After the initial neurological adaptations, there starts to be a noticeable increase in muscle mass. This is due to hypertrophy of the individual muscle fibers through increases in cytoplasmic volume, myofibrils, and contractile protein filaments. Muscle fiber hypertrophy has been reported to be greater in fast-twitch fibers than slow-twitch fibers, but most research studies do not support this finding.

The increase in muscle mass may also be caused by hyperplasia (an increase in the number of muscle fibers). Although hyperplasia has not been directly demonstrated in humans, it has been demonstrated to occur in the muscle of experimental animals taught to lift weights for rewards. It has also been observed that the muscle fiber sizes of some strength athletes are the same as those of individuals of average size and muscle mass. Clearly, an increase in fiber number is the only way to account for the increase in muscle mass of these strength athletes. However, an increase in muscle mass due to hyperplasia is probably difficult to achieve and requires many years of training.

The metabolic adaptations that occur with resistance training are small compared with endurance training. There are small increases in the activities of the glycolytic enzymes and the enzymes that rapidly restore ATP. There are also small increases in the ATP and CP stores. If the training program results in high muscle and blood lactic acid accumulation, there is also an increase in muscle proteins that buffer or neutralize the lactic acid, and increase lactic acid tolerance and muscle endurance. However, there may also be a reduced capillary and mitochondrial density with resistance training. This is the result of a dilution of these structures due to an increase in the size of the muscle fibers. This means that individuals who only resistance-train may risk decreasing their aerobic endurance.

Table 12.3 summarizes the different adaptations that occur with endurance and resistance training.

Mechanism of Muscle Adaptation

Muscle fibers are approximately 20 percent protein and it is the protein that determines their physiologic and metabolic characteristics. By increasing, decreasing, or modifying the protein content, the functionality of the muscle can be changed. In actuality, the proteins that comprise the muscle fiber are constantly being synthesized and destroyed. This flux is called "protein turnover". When synthesis equals degradation, the protein content doesn't change. However when synthesis exceeds degradation protein content is increased and when degradation exceeds synthesis protein content is reduced.

TABLE 12.3. Training Adaptations	
Endurance Adaptations	**Resistance Adaptations**
Increase in heart weight	Increase in tendon and ligament strength
Increase in heart size	Greater coordination of muscle fiber recruitment
Increase in the number of blood vessels around each muscle fiber	Increase in the number of muscle fibers
Increase in size and number of muscle mitochondria	Increase in size of individual fibers
Increase in the lactate threshold	Increase in the activities of enzymes that restore ATP
Increase in proteins that control glucose uptake and glycogen storage	Increase in ATP and CP stores
	Increase in lactic acid tolerance
	Reduction in the number of blood vessels and mitochondria per muscle fiber

Muscle fibers are highly adaptable. This is because the genes of the muscle are very responsive to both extracellular stimuli such as hormones and intracellular stimuli such as the level of ATP. Altering the expression of specific genes is the basis for the adaptive responses that occur as a result of strength training. By altering gene expression, rates of synthesis and degradation can be altered to increase or decrease the level of a specific protein in the muscle fiber.

To appreciate how training and nutrition work together to bring about muscle adaptations specific to exercise performed, you must first understand how the genetic machinery of the muscle functions. An increase in the level of a specific protein can be controlled at three different levels (see Figure 12.2 on page 160).

The first level is gene transcription. Genes that hold the information on how a protein is manufactured are located on specific sites on the muscle's DNA. When a gene is activated, it will replicate the information in the form of a blueprint called messenger RNA. A number of stimuli can activate a gene including hormones, the energy state of the muscle (amount of ATP and creatine phosphate, or CP) and even levels of different nutrients.

The second level of control is protein translation. During translation, the messenger RNA in combination with small protein assembly plants called ribosomes, assemble amino acids in the sequence specified by the messenger RNA to form a designated protein. When the ribosomes complete their mission, protein translation stops. Hormones such as insulin and the availability of amino acids are two of the control factors that positively influence protein translation.

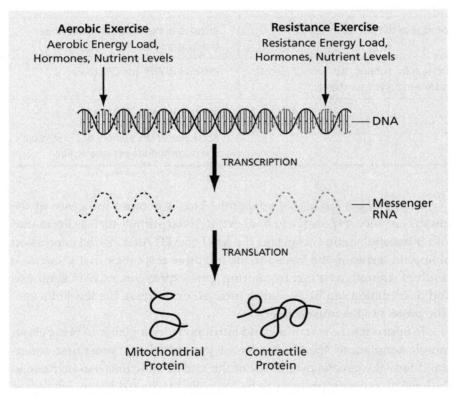

Figure 12.2. Impact of Exercise Type on Gene Expression
Depending on the type of exercise, genes for different proteins are activated. When the gene is activated, it causes the release of a specific messenger RNA molecule, which serves as a blueprint for the assembly of a specific protein by ribosomes, which are essentailly protein assembly plants. Aerobic exercise, for example, can increase the number of mitochondrial proteins, and resistance exercise can increase the number of contractile proteins.

For example, after exercise the muscle is very sensitive to the activation of protein translation by amino acids (metabolic sensitivity) and the hormone insulin. Consuming a carbohydrate/protein drink (nutrient activation) immediately after exercise increases insulin levels, amino acid availability, and promotes ribosome assembly. The net result is an increase in protein synthesis. Although exercise stimulates the actual gene transcription, nutrient intervention at the right time results in a higher rate of protein synthesis.

The third level of control, protein degradation, is less well understood. It is known that exercise stimulates and insulin inhibits protein degradation. Biolo and colleagues from the University of Texas Health Science Center in Galveston demonstrated that following exercise, protein synthesis was increased but so was protein degradation resulting in a net protein loss. When insulin levels were increased, protein degradation was reduced, resulting in a net protein gain. These results show that whether protein is gained or lost after exercise depends on the rates of both protein synthesis and protein degradation. It also reemphasizes that nutritional intervention, in this case via insulin, can shift the equation in the anabolic direction.

SUMMARY

Muscle is made up of bundles of muscle fibers called fasciculi. There are two basic types of muscle fibers, slow twitch and fast twitch. The physiological and metabolic characteristics of the slow- and fast-twitch fibers differ, which allows for a more diverse performance capability. Muscle is a highly adaptable tissue but the adaptations that occur with training are specific to the type, intensity, and duration of training. While exercise provides a strong stimulus for adaptation, the rate of adaptation can be strongly influenced by nutrient availability. It should be clear that the combination of exercise and nutrient supplementation can have a strong influence on protein synthesis and muscle tissue development.

KEY TAKEAWAYS

- Skeletal muscle is composed of slow-twitch and fast-twitch muscle fibers, which have different physiological and metabolic characteristics.

- Speed and force of muscle contraction are determined by the number and types of muscle fibers (slow-twitch or fast-twitch) activated, and by the frequency of their activation.

- Muscle adaptation is very specific to the type, intensity, and duration of training.

- Make your workout program specific to the physical adaptations you seek through training (for example, if you seek explosive power, incorporate some high-speed lifts).

- Incorporate into your workout program the four basic principles of exercise training.

- The two primary adaptations to resistance training are hypertrophy of individual muscle fibers and synchronization of muscle-fiber recruitment.

- Although genetics play an important role in muscle cell adaptation, the process can be significantly influenced by nutritional intervention.

- Customize your training to account for your genetic strengths and weaknesses.

Conclusion

When the first studies on the importance of Nutrient Timing were published, they were met with skepticism by many exercise physiologists and nutritionists. There have now been many studies conducted worldwide in the laboratories of respected researchers that support the science underlying Nutrient Timing. This does not mean that we have all the information we need. Additional studies are essential if we are to fully understand and elucidate the mechanisms by which nutrition can influence muscle cell growth and development. However, it is also clear that the science as of this moment strongly supports the premise that strength athletes, and, in fact, all athletes, trainers, strength and conditioning coaches, and nutritionists will benefit by incorporating the principles of Nutrient Timing into their programs.

In the last few years, we have seen sports nutrition dominated by the use of illegal drugs and supplements. However, the many studies we have cited show that Nutrient Timing gives us a tool which will enable athletes to safely achieve gains in strength, power, and performance with the most basic of all tools—the food they eat.

We anticipate further exciting breakthroughs as we watch the science of Nutrient Timing continue to develop.

Glossary

Actin. One of the two major contractile proteins in muscle cells. *See also* Myosin.

Activation. *See* Nutrient activation.

Adaptation. A physiological or biochemical change that occurs when the body is exposed to repeated bouts of exercise.

Adenosine triphosphate (ATP). *See* ATP.

Adrenaline. *See* Epinephrine.

Aerobic metabolism. The process of energy production (ATP) that occurs in the mitochondria and requires the presence of oxygen.

Agonist. A muscle that initiates and is primarily responsible for movement.

Alpha-lipoic acid. An enzyme cofactor in the conversion of glucose into energy; also an antioxidant.

Amino acids. The biochemical building blocks of proteins. There are twenty amino acids, eleven of which are nonessential and can be manufactured by the body, and nine of which are essential and cannot be manufactured by the body, so they must be supplied through diet.

Anabolic. The building up of body tissue and fuel stores.

Anabolic Phase. The second phase of nutrient timing, occurring within the first forty-five minutes after a resistance workout, during which acute muscle recovery occurs.

Anaerobic metabolism. The process by which energy is produced that does not require the presence of oxygen.

Anaerobic threshold. The exercise intensity beyond which lactic acid begins to rapidly accumulate in the working muscles, hastening exhaustion.

Antagonist. A muscle or muscle group that opposes muscle contraction.

Antioxidant. A substance that neutralizes free radicals and prevents tissue damage.

Asynchronous. Refers to a muscle movement pattern wherein motor units are recruited in a sequential pattern that allows for rest periods between contractions. Asynchronous contraction patterns are characteristic of sustained, low-intensity to moderately high-intensity movements (for example, jogging).

ATP. Adenosine triphosphate; a high-energy compound that is the fundamental source of energy for muscle contractions.

ATPase. An enzyme that breaks down ATP to release energy.

Autogenic inhibition. A reflex inhibition of motor neuron discharge that occurs to prevent excessive muscle tension, which can cause damage to muscle and its connective tissues.

Branched-chain amino acids (BCAAs). Essential amino acids that inhibit muscle protein breakdown and aid in muscle glycogen storage. The BCAAs are valine, leucine, and isoleucine.

Calcium. A metallic element that is an essential nutrient for humans. It is the main structural ingredient of bones and plays an essential role in muscle contractions.

Calorie. A unit of energy-producing potential that is contained in food and released during aerobic metabolism.

Capillaries. Tiny blood vessels that allow for the exchange of gases and nutrients between blood and tissue cells.

Carbohydrate. A broad category of organic compounds that are contained in food and serve as a major energy source in the body, especially during exercise.

Casein. A high-quality protein that is a product of the cheese-making process.

Catabolism. The process of breaking down the body tissues, particularly skeletal muscle.

Cellular respiration. *See* Aerobic metabolism.

Cellulose. A dietary fiber that is contained in plant foods and aids the human digestion and excretion processes.

Coenzyme Q_{10} (CoQ_{10}). A powerful antioxidant that protects the body from free radicals.

Complete protein. A protein that contains all nine essential amino acids.

Complex carbohydrates (polysaccharides). A carbohydrate made from three or more simple sugar molecules. The two major categories of complex carbohydrates are starches and fibers.

Concentric. Refers to a type of muscle contraction wherein the muscle shortens as it contracts.

Cortisol. A catabolic hormone that breaks down muscle proteins for use as an energy source. It is released during strenuous exercise or when blood glucose drops below normal levels.

Creatine monohydrate. A form of creatine that is taken as a dietary supplement in order to increase creatine phosphate storage in the muscles.

Creatine phosphate (CP). A high-energy compound that is stored in muscle cells in small amounts and provides a quick energy source for high-intensity anaerobic exercise or work.

Cytoplasm. The fluid medium inside a cell.

Dehydration. A state in which the amount of water in the body has diminished below the level needed for optimal athletic performance.

Disuse. An exercise principle, which states that the body will quickly lose adaptations to previous exercise training if training is discontinued.

Eccentric. Refers to a type of muscle contraction wherein the muscle lengthens as it contracts, as for example, the lengthening of the biceps during the lowering phase of a biceps curl.

Economy. The relative energy efficiency of a swimmer, cyclist, or runner in motion. It refers to the amount of energy an athlete requires to travel at a given pace as compared to other athletes.

Electrolytes. Mineral nutrients (sodium, chloride, magnesium, and potassium) that aid muscle contraction, nerve impulse transmission, and other biochemical processes.

Endurance. The ability to sustain work or resist fatigue.

Energy Phase. The workout, or during-exercise, phase of the Nutrient Timing System.

Enzyme. A protein that promotes one or more types of chemical reaction in the body without itself being altered.

Epinephrine. A hormone that stimulates liver and muscle glycogen breakdown, lipolysis, and gluconeogenesis.

Ergogenic aid. Anything that enhances physical performance. Sports drinks and energy bars and gels are considered ergogenic aids.

Ergolytic. Anything that will impair physical performance.

Fascicule. A bundle of muscle fibers within a muscle.

Fast-twitch muscle fiber. The type of muscle fiber best suited to anaerobic energy production. Also called type II muscle fibers.

Fatigue. The inability to continue to work or exercise.

Fatty acid. The components of fat that are used by the body for energy.

Free radicals. Highly reactive chemicals that damage body tissues by pilfering electrons in order to improve their own stability.

Fructose. Known as "fruit sugar" because it is the type of sugar that is most abundant in fruit. It is sweeter and not as easily digested as glucose.

Glucagon. A hormone that stimulates liver glycogen breakdown, gluconeogenesis, and lipolysis.

Gluconeogenesis. A biochemical process by which small three-carbon compounds such as lactate and some amino acids are converted into glucose by the liver. Gluconeogenesis is increased to maintain blood glucose levels.

Glucose. A simple sugar derived from the breakdown of dietary carbohydrate that serves as a major energy fuel.

Glutamine. The most abundant amino acid in the body; especially abundant in skeletal muscles. Glutamine can be converted to glucose and used for energy and is also important for immune function.

Glycemic index. A measure of how different foods affect blood glucose levels relative to ingestion of pure glucose.

Glycogen. The form in which glucose is stored in the muscle and liver.

Glycolysis. One of two forms of anaerobic energy production, in which glycogen is metabolized without oxygen. Also referred to as the "glycolytic pathway."

Glycolytic pathway. The enzymatic pathway in the cell where glycolysis takes place.

Growth hormone. An anabolic hormone secreted by the pituitary gland that stimulates bone and connective tissue growth and lipolysis.

Growth Phase. The third phase of the Nutrient Timing System, which begins about forty-five minutes after completion of exercise (that is, after the Anabolic Phase) and ends ten minutes prior to the subsequent workout.

Hemoglobin. An oxygen-binding protein in red blood cells that transports oxygen in the circulatory system.

High-quality protein. A type of protein that scores high on any of the four scientific measures of protein quality, which rate the effects of proteins in the body.

HMB (beta-hydroxybeta methlbutyrate). A compound that is produced in the body from the essential amino acid leucine; it prevents muscle protein breakdown.

Homeostasis. A state of balance, or equilibrium, in a given system of the body.

Hyperglycemia. A state wherein the blood glucose level is above normal.

Hyperplasia. Muscle growth resulting from an increase in the number of muscle fibers.

Hypertrophy. Muscle growth resulting from an increase in the size of muscle fibers.

Hypoglycemia. A state wherein the blood glucose level is too low to support normal functioning of the body.

Incomplete protein. A protein that does not contain one or more of the essential amino acids.

Insulin. A hormone that is secreted by the pancreas; it stimulates the transport of glucose and amino acids into muscle and promotes glycogen storage and protein synthesis.

Insulin-like growth factors. Proteins that are produced in the body. They mimic many of the functions of the hormone insulin.

Insulin resistance. When the muscle's response to insulin is less than normal.

Insulin sensitivity. Describes the manner in which the muscle responds to insulin. A decrease in insulin sensitivity is the same as an increase in insulin resistance, whereas an increase in insulin sensitivity means the muscle response is greater than normal.

Intensity. The rate at which energy is used relative to the muscle mass recruited.

Iron. An essential trace mineral that is involved in the formation of the blood compound hemoglobin and the transportation of oxygen.

Isometric. Refers to a type of muscle contraction wherein muscle tension the length of the muscle does not change (that is, no movement is produced).

Lactate threshold. An intensity level of exercise above which the metabolic waste product lactic acid accumulates in the blood faster than the circulatory system can remove it. Also known as the "anaerobic threshold."

Lactic acid (lactate). A byproduct of anaerobic metabolism and a fuel for aerobic metabolism and gluconeogenesis.

L-Carnitine. A vitamin-like nutrient that helps the body release energy from fat.

Lipolysis. The breakdown of stored fats to free fatty acids.

Low-quality protein. A type of protein that scores lower than most other types of protein on the four scientific measures of protein quality.

Macronutrients. The three essential nutrient types (excluding water) that are present in great abundance in the body: carbohydrate, fatty acids (that is, fat), and protein.

Maltodextrin. A complex carbohydrate that is used in many ergogenic aids (sports drinks, carbohydrate gels, and energy bars) because it is easily digested.

Medium-chain triglycerides (MTC). A class of fatty acids that are rapidly absorbed and burned as energy.

Messenger RNA. A form of RNA that transfers genetic information from the cell nucleus to ribosomes in the cell cytoplasm.

Metabolic sensitivity. Refers to the muscles' ability to quickly change their function in response to various stimuli.

Mitochondria. Structures within cells that serve as the site of aerobic metabolism.

Muscle fiber. A long, thin, single cell within a muscle that is capable of contracting to produce force.

Muscular endurance. The ability of the muscle to avoid fatigue.

Myocardium. The scientific name for the heart muscle.

Myofibril. A chain of sarcomeres within a muscle fiber.

Myoglobin. An oxygen-carrying compound similar to hemoglobin but found in muscle.

Myosin. One of two major contractile proteins within muscle cells. *See also* Actin.

Norepinephrine. A hormone that stimulates heart rate and metabolic reactions such as lipolysis and gluconeogenesis. Also called noradrenaline.

Nucleotides. The building blocks of nucleic acids, which include DNA, the genetic "blueprint" molecule, and ATP, the most fundamental energy source for muscular activity.

Nutrient activation. A process by which one type of nutrient enhances the effects of a second type of nutrient.

Nutrient optimization. Refers to the ability of muscles to shift from a catabolic to an anabolic state because of the availability of key nutrients.

Periodization. Varying the training stimulus over discrete periods of time to prevent overtraining.

Phosphagen pathway. One of two forms of anaerobic energy systems, in which adenosine triphosphate (ATP) is resynthesized by the energy released from the breakdown of creatine phosphate.

Placebo. An inactive substance usually provided in a manner identical to an active substance, to test for real versus imagined effects.

Power. The product of force and velocity.

Prime mover. A muscle that bears the heaviest workload in a given movement pattern.

Progressive overload. The practice of stimulating physical adaptations to exercise by consistently requiring the body to work slightly harder than it is used to working.

Protein. The fundamental structural components of all living cells and many bioactive substances such as enzymes, hormones, and antibodies. Proteins are composed of amino acids.

Protein accretion. An increase in the protein concentration within a muscle.

Protein turnover. The combination of protein synthesis and protein degradation.

Recovery. A process wherein one or more systems of the body return to homeostasis following exertion.

Ribose. A simple sugar found in cells. It is involved in the production of nucleotides, which are needed to produce ATP.

Ribosome. A particle made of ribose and protein that is found in the cytoplasm of living cells and serves as the assembly site for polypeptides encoded by messenger RNA.

Sarcomere. The smallest functional unit of a muscle fiber, which consists of the major contractile proteins myosin and actin.

Simple carbohydrate. A carbohydrate with a relatively basic molecular structure.

Slow-twitch muscle fiber. A type of muscle fiber that is better able to produce energy aerobically than anaerobically. Also called type I muscle fiber.

Soy protein. A type of protein contained in or derived from soybeans.

Specificity. An exercise principle which states that the body will adapt in response to the specific demands placed upon it in an exercise program.

Strength. The ability of a muscle to exert force.

Sucrose. Ordinary table sugar. A common ingredient in sports drinks because it is quickly metabolized to provide fast energy.

Sugar. Another name for a simple carbohydrate.

Synchronous. Refers to a muscle movement pattern wherein large numbers of individual fibers contract simultaneously to produce strong forces. Synchronous fiber recruitment patterns are characteristic of high-intensity movements (for example, weightlifting).

Synergist. A muscle that plays a secondary role in generating a certain movement.

Tendon. A strong sheath of connective tissue that connects a muscle to a bone.

Testosterone. A hormone that is responsible for many secondary male sexual characteristics and also facilitates muscle growth.

Transcription. The process of transferring genetic information from the DNA to messenger RNA.

Translation. The assembly of amino acids into polypeptides according to instructions provided by the messenger RNA.

Type I muscle fiber. *See* Slow-twitch muscle fiber.

Type II muscle fiber. *See* Fast-twitch muscle fiber.

Vitamin. Any of a number of fat-soluble or water-soluble organic substances obtained from plant and animal foods that are essential for normal biological functioning.

VO$_2$ max. The maximum rate at which a given athlete can consume oxygen. The higher an athlete's VO$_2$ max, the faster he or she can run, swim, bike, and so on without accumulating excess lactic acid in the working muscles.

Whey protein. A source of amino acids derived from milk.

Appendix A

Caloric Expenditure Calculator

To determine your average Daily Caloric Expenditure (DCE), you first have to determine your Resting Caloric Expenditure (RCE), Daily Activities Caloric Expenditure (DA), and Workout Caloric Expenditure (WCE). Once you have these figures, you will add them together to determine your DCE.

1. Resting Caloric Expenditure (RCE)

Resting Caloric Expenditure (RCE) is determined as follows:

- For men, RCE = body weight (in pounds) x 11 calories per pound
- For women, RCE = body weight (in pounds) x 10 calories per pound

  For example, the RCE for a 200-pound man equals 2,200 calories (200 pounds x 11 calories per pound).

Body weight (in pounds) _____ x _____ calories = **your RCE:** _____

2. Daily Activities Caloric Expenditure (DA)

Daily Activities Caloric Expenditure (DA) is determined from the appropriate percentage in Table A.1 on page 175 and from the above RCE figure.

- DA = RCE x "Percentage of RCE" from Table A.1

  For example, a 200-pound store clerk's DA is 990 calories (2,200 RCE x 45 percent [or 0.45] = 990 calories [DA])

RCE (above) _____ x _____ % of RCE (Table A.1) = **your DA:** _____

TABLE A.1. Daily Activity Levels and Resting Caloric Expenditure

	Percentage of RCE	
DAILY ACTIVITY LEVEL	Men	Women
Sedentary Sits most of the day (for example, computer programmer, business person, secretary)	15%	15%
Lightly active Walks or stands most of the day (for example, teacher, homemaker, delivery person)	35%	30%
Moderately active Walks and performs some light physical labor (for example, mechanic, store clerk, machinist)	45%	40%
Very active Has a physically active job (for example, landscaper, laborer, dancer, steelworker, construction worker, farmer)	75%	70%
Exceptionally active Has a very physically active job (for example, lumberjack, wilderness guide, miner)	100%	90%

3. Workout Caloric Expenditure (WCE)

Your Workout Caloric Expenditure (WCE) is determined from the appropriate figure in Table A.2 on page 176 multiplied by your body weight and workout time. Determine your (WCE) as follows:

- WCE = Caloric Expenditure (from Table A.2) x your body weight (in pounds) x workout time (see below)

DETERMINING YOUR ACTUAL WORKOUT TIME

The exercise intensities in Table A.2 are based on thirty-second sets with a forty-five-second rest period between sets. Therefore, to determine your actual workout time, multiply the total number of sets completed (total sets = number of exercises x sets per exercise) by 1.25 minutes (30 second set + 45 second rest).

For example, our 200-pound man's exercise program is high intensity (0.058 cal/lb/min) and composed of exercises of three sets each, so his workout time is (10 x 3) x 1.25 minutes or 37.5 minutes.

Knowing his actual workout time, we calculate his WCE as follows:

• WCE = 0.058 cal/lb/min x 200 lb x 37.5 min = 435

Caloric Expenditure (Table A.2) _____ x Body Weight (in pounds) _____

x Workout Time (see above) _____ = **your WCE:** _____

Table A.2 lists the caloric expenditures at five different exercise intensities. To determine your Workout Caloric Expenditure, use the figure that best represents your workout.

TABLE A.2. Exercise Intensity and Caloric Expenditure		
	Caloric Expenditure (calories per pound per minute)	
EXERCISE INTENSITY	Men	Women
Circuit Training, 15 reps/exercise	0.053	0.045
Low (60%) 1RM, 10 reps/set	0.048	0.042
Moderate (70%) 1RM, 10 reps/set	0.055	0.048
High (75%) 1RM, 8 reps/set	0.058	0.055
Intense (80%) 1RM, 5 reps/set	0.061	0.058

4. Daily Caloric Expenditure (DCE)

To figure your DCE, add your RCE to your DA and WCE.

For example, our 200-pound man's Daily Caloric Expenditure = 2,200 (RCE) + 990 (DA) + 435 (WCE) or 3,625 calories.

Your RCE _____ + DA _____ + WCE _____ = **your DCE:** _____

Appendix B

Meal Plan Templates

The following Meal Plan Templates are designed to help you create your personal NTS Nutrition Plan.

1 Determine your daily caloric intake using the Caloric Expenditure Calculator in Appendix A.

2 Select the meal plan template that is closest to your calorie needs. The meal plan templates are designed to deliver a daily protein content of 1.14 grams of protein per pound of body weight.

3 Refer to Table 8.1 on page 93 to personalize your diet. Select foods from this table and fill them into the templates.

If your calories needs are slightly different from those listed in the templates, do the following:

1 Determine your daily caloric intake using the Caloric Expenditure Calculator in Appendix A.

2 Distribute your calories as follows: 24 percent protein, 43 percent carbohydrate, and 33 percent fat.

3 Adjust the protein, carbohydrate, and fat percentages in the template by adding or subtracting foods according to their individual nutrient contents listed in Table 8.1. Select foods from this table to personalize your diet.

Daily Food Group Template 1

PROFILE: Female 130 lbs • 18 calories per pound • GOAL: 2,340 calories

	Servings	Protein	Carbs	Fat	Cal
Starch	3	9	45	3	243
Fruit	5	—	75	—	300
Milk	2	16	24	2	178
Added Sugars	2	—	8	—	32
Vegetables	5	10	25	—	140
Meat/Meat Substitutes					
Very Lean	3	21	—	—	84
Lean	3	21	—	9	165
Med Fat	3	21	—	15	219
Fat	11	—	—	55	495
NTS Energy Supplement	1	6	24	1	129
NTS Anabolic Supplement	1	15	45	1	249
NTS Growth Supplement	1	20	4	1	105
Total Grams		139	250	87	
Daily Calories		556	1,000	783	2,339
Nutrient Composition		24%	43%	33%	

Sample Food Menu Plan 1

	Food Group	Servings	Protein	Carb	Fat	Cal
Breakfast	Starch	1	3	15	1	81
	Fruit	2	—	30	—	120
	Milk	1	8	12	1	89
	Fat	1	—	—	5	45
Breakfast Total			11	57	7	335

Workout	NTS Energy Supplement	1	6	24	1	129
Immediately Post-workout	NTS Anabolic Supplement	1	15	45	1	249
2 Hours Post-workout	NTS Growth Supplement	1	20	4	1	105
Lunch	Starch	1	3	15	1	81
	Fruit	2	—	30	—	120
	Vegetables	2	4	10	—	56
	Med Fat	3	21	—	15	219
	Fat	3	—	—	15	135
Lunch Total			28	55	31	611
Snack	Milk	1	8	12	1	89
	Added Sugars	2	—	8	—	32
	Fat	3	—	—	15	135
Snack Total			8	20	16	256
Dinner	Starch	1	3	15	1	81
	Fruit	1	—	15	—	60
	Vegetables	3	6	15	—	84
	Very Lean	3	21	—	—	84
	Lean	3	21	—	9	165
	Fat	4	—	—	20	180
Dinner Total			51	45	30	654
Total (Actual)			139	250	87	2,339

Daily Food Group Template 2

PROFILE: Female 145 lbs • 18 calories per pound • GOAL: 2,610 calories

	Total	Protein	Carbs	Fat	Cal
Starch	4	12	60	4	324
Fruit	5	—	75	—	300
Milk	2	16	24	2	178
Added Sugars	4	—	16	—	64
Vegetables	5	10	25	—	140
Meat/Meat Substitutes					
Very Lean	6	42	—	—	168
Lean	4	28	—	12	220
Med Fat	2	14	—	10	146
Fat	13	—	—	65	585
NTS Energy Supplement	1	6	24	1	129
NTS Anabolic Supplement	1	15	45	1	249
NTS Growth Supplement	1	20	4	1	105
Total Grams		163	273	96	
Daily Calories		652	1,092	864	2,608
Nutrient Composition		25%	42%	33%	

Sample Food Menu Plan 2

	Food Group	Servings	Protein	Carb	Fat	Cal
Breakfast	Starch	1	3	15	1	81
	Fruit	2	—	30	—	120
	Milk	1	8	12	1	89
	Added Sugars	1	—	4	—	16

	Med Fat	2	14	—	10	146
	Fat	2	—	—	10	90
Breakfast Total			25	61	22	542
Workout	NTS Energy Supplement	1	6	24	1	129
Immediately Post-workout	NTS Anabolic Supplement	1	15	45	1	249
2 Hours Post-workout	NTS Growth Supplement	1	20	4	1	105
Lunch	Starch	2	6	30	2	162
	Fruit	2	—	30	—	120
	Vegetables	2	4	10	—	56
	Lean	4	28	—	12	220
	Fat	3	—	—	15	135
Lunch Total			38	70	29	693
Snack	Milk	1	8	12	1	89
	Added Sugars	3	—	12	—	48
	Fat	4	—	—	20	180
Snack Total			8	24	21	317
Dinner	Starch	1	3	15	1	81
	Fruit	1	—	15	—	60
	Vegetables	3	6	15	—	84
	Very Lean	6	42	—	—	168
	Fat	4	—	—	20	180
Dinner Total			51	45	21	573
Total (Actual)			163	273	96	2,608

Daily Food Group Template 3

PROFILE: Male 160 lbs • 19 calories per pound • GOAL: 3,040 calories

	Total	Protein	Carbs	Fat	Cal
Starch	7	21	105	7	567
Fruit	4	—	60	—	240
Milk	2	16	24	2	178
Added Sugars	8	—	32	—	128
Vegetables	6	12	30	—	168
Meat/Meat Substitutes					
Very Lean	3	21	—	—	84
Lean	5	35	—	15	275
Med Fat	2	14	—	10	146
Fat	15	—	—	75	675
NTS Energy Supplement	1	6	24	1	129
NTS Anabolic Supplement	1	15	45	1	249
NTS Growth Supplement	2	40	8	2	210
Total Grams		180	328	113	
Daily Calories		720	1,312	1,017	3,049
Nutrient Composition		24%	43%	33%	

Sample Food Menu Plan 3

	Food Group	Servings	Protein	Carb	Fat	Cal
Breakfast	Starch	2	6	30	2	162
	Fruit	1	—	15	—	60
	Milk	1	8	12	1	89
	Added Sugars	3	—	12	—	48

	Vegetables	2	4	10	—	56
	Med Fat	2	14	—	10	146
	Fat	3	—	—	15	135
Breakfast Total			32	79	28	696
Workout	NTS Energy Supplement	1	6	24	1	129
Immediately Post-workout	NTS Anabolic Supplement	1	15	45	1	249
2 Hours Post-workout	NTS Growth Supplement	1	20	4	1	105
Lunch	Starch	2	6	30	2	162
	Fruit	1	—	15	—	60
	Very Lean	3	21	—	—	84
	Fat	4	—	—	20	180
Lunch Total			48	45	22	570
Snack	Starch	2	6	30	2	162
	Fruit	1	—	15	—	60
	Milk	1	8	12	1	89
	Added Sugars	5	—	20	—	80
	Fat	4	—	—	20	180
Snack Total			14	81	23	587
Dinner	Starch	1	3	15	1	81
	Fruit	1	—	15	—	60
	Vegetables	4	8	20	—	112
	Lean	5	35	—	15	275
	Fat	4	—	—	20	180
Dinner Total			46	50	36	708
Post Dinner	NTS Growth Supplement	1	20	4	1	105
Total (Actual)			180	328	113	3,049

Daily Food Group Template 4

PROFILE: Male 180 lbs • 19 calories per pound • GOAL: 3,420 calories

	Total	Protein	Carbs	Fat	Cal
Starch	7	21	105	7	567
Fruit	6	—	90	—	360
Milk	2	16	24	2	178
Added Sugars	9	—	36	—	144
Vegetables	6	12	30	—	168
Meat/Meat Substitutes					
Very Lean	6	42	—	—	168
Lean	6	42	—	18	330
Med Fat	2	14	—	10	146
Fat	17	—	—	85	765
NTS Energy Supplement	1	6	24	1	129
NTS Anabolic Supplement	1	15	45	1	249
NTS Growth Supplement	2	40	8	2	210
Total Grams		208	362	126	
Daily Calories		832	1,448	1,134	3,414
Nutrient Composition		24%	42%	33%	

Sample Food Menu Plan 4

	Food Group	Servings	Protein	Carb	Fat	Cal
Breakfast	Starch	2	6	30	2	162
	Fruit	2	—	30	—	120
	Milk	1	8	12	1	89
	Added Sugars	3	—	12	—	48
	Med Fat	2	14	—	10	146

	Fat	2	—	—	10	90
Breakfast Total			28	84	23	655
Workout	NTS Energy Supplement	1	6	24	1	129
Immediately Post-workout	NTS Anabolic Supplement	1	15	45	1	249
2 Hours Post-workout	NTS Growth Supplement	1	20	4	1	105
Lunch	Starch	2	6	30	2	162
	Fruit	2	—	30	—	120
	Vegetables	2	4	10	—	56
	Very Lean	6	42	—	—	168
	Fat	3	—	—	15	135
Lunch Total			52	70	17	641
Snack	Starch	2	6	30	2	162
	Milk	1	8	12	1	89
	Added Sugars	6	—	24	—	96
	Fat	6	—	—	30	270
Snack Total			14	66	33	617
Dinner	Starch	1	3	15	1	81
	Fruit	2	—	30	—	120
	Vegetables	4	8	20	—	112
	Lean	6	42	—	18	330
	Fat	6	—	—	30	270
Dinner Total			53	65	49	913
Post Dinner	NTS Growth Supplement	1	20	4	1	105
Total (Actual)			208	362	126	3,414

Daily Food Group Template 5

PROFILE: Male 200 lbs • 19 calories per pound • GOAL: 3,800 calories

	Total	Protein	Carbs	Fat	Cal
Starch	8	24	120	8	648
Fruit	8	—	120	—	480
Milk	3	24	36	3	267
Added Sugars	7	—	28	—	11
Vegetables	6	12	30	—	168
Meat/Meat Substitutes					
Very Lean	7	49	—	—	196
Lean	6	42	—	18	330
Med Fat	2	14	—	10	146
Fat	19	—	—	95	855
NTS Energy Supplement	1	6	24	1	129
NTS Anabolic Supplement	1	15	45	1	249
NTS Growth Supplement	2	40	8	2	210
Total Grams		226	411	138	
Daily Calories		904	1,644	1,242	3,790
Nutrient Composition		23%	43%	33%	

Sample Food Menu Plan 5

	Food Group	Servings	Protein	Carb	Fat	Cal
Breakfast	Starch	2	6	30	2	162
	Fruit	2	—	30	—	120
	Milk	1	8	12	1	89
	Added Sugars	2	—	12	—	32
	Med Fat	3	21	—	15	219
	Fat	3	—	—	15	135

Breakfast Total			**28**	**80**	**28**	**684**
Workout	NTS Energy Supplement	I	6	24	I	129
Immediately Post-workout	NTS Anabolic Supplement	I	15	45	I	249
2 Hours Post-workout	NTS Growth Supplement	I	20	4	I	105
Lunch	Starch	2	6	30	2	162
	Fruit	2	—	30	—	120
	Milk	I	8	12	I	89
	Vegetables	2	4	10	—	56
	Very Lean	4	28	—	—	112
	Lean	2	14	—	6	110
	Fat	3	—	—	15	135
Lunch Total			**60**	**82**	**24**	**784**
Snack	Starch	2	6	30	2	162
	Fruit	2	—	30	—	120
	Milk	I	8	12	I	89
	Added Sugars	5	—	20	—	80
	Fat	6	—	—	30	270
Snack Total			**14**	**92**	**33**	**721**
Dinner	Starch	2	6	30	2	162
	Fruit	2	—	30	—	120
	Vegetables	4	8	20	—	112
	Very Lean	2	14	—	—	56
	Lean	4	28	—	12	220
	Fat	7	—	—	35	315
Dinner Total			**63**	**80**	**49**	**1,013**
Post Dinner	NTS Growth Supplement	I	20	4	I	105
Total (Actual)			**226**	**411**	**138**	**3,790**

Daily Food Group Template 6

PROFILE: Male 225 lbs • 19 calories per pound • GOAL: 4,275 calories

	Total	Protein	Carbs	Fat	Cal
Starch	10	30	150	10	810
Fruit	8	—	120	—	480
Milk	3	24	36	3	267
Added Sugars	13	—	52	—	208
Vegetables	6	12	30	—	168
Meat/Meat Substitutes					
Very Lean	6	42	—	—	168
Lean	9	63	—	27	495
Med Fat	3	21	—	15	219
Fat	19	—	—	95	855
NTS Energy Supplement	1	6	24	1	129
NTS Anabolic Supplement	1	15	45	1	249
NTS Growth Supplement	2	40	8	2	210
Total Grams		253	465	154	
Daily Calories		1,012	1,860	1,386	4,258
Nutrient Composition		24%	44%	33%	

Sample Food Menu Plan 6

	Food Group	Servings	Protein	Carb	Fat	Cal
Breakfast	Starch	2	6	30	2	162
	Fruit	2	—	30	—	120
	Milk	1	8	12	1	89
	Added Sugars	4	—	16	—	64
	Very Lean	1	7	—	—	28
	Med Fat	2	14	—	10	146
	Fat	3	—	—	15	135

Breakfast Total			**35**	**88**	**28**	**744**
Workout	NTS Energy Supplement	I	6	24	I	129
Immediately Post-workout	NTS Anabolic Supplement	I	15	45	I	249
2 Hours Post-workout	NTS Growth Supplement	I	20	4	I	105
Lunch	Starch	3	9	45	3	243
	Fruit	2	—	30	—	120
	Milk	I	8	12	I	89
	Added Sugars	3	—	12	—	48
	Vegetables	2	4	10	—	56
	Very Lean	5	35	—	—	140
	Lean	3	21	—	9	165
	Med Fat	I	7	—	5	73
	Fat	4	—	—	20	180
Lunch Total			**84**	**109**	**38**	**1,114**
Snack	Starch	2	6	30	2	162
	Fruit	2	—	30	—	120
	Milk	I	8	12	I	89
	Added Sugars	6	—	24	—	96
	Fat	5	—	—	25	225
Snack Total			**14**	**96**	**28**	**692**
Dinner	Starch	3	9	45	3	243
	Fruit	2	—	30	—	120
	Vegetables	4	8	20	—	112
	Lean	6	42	—	18	330
	Fat	7	—	—	35	315
Dinner Total			**59**	**95**	**56**	**1,120**
Post Dinner	NTS Growth Sup	I	20	4	I	105
Total (Actual)			**253**	**465**	**154**	**4,258**

Bibliography

Chapter 1: Nutrient Timing

Biolo, G., Tipton, K.D., Klein, S., et al., "An abundant supply of amino acids enhances the metabolic effect of exercise on muscle protein," *American Journal of Physiology*, 273: E122–E119, 1997.

Gleeson, M., Lancaster, G.I., and Bishop, N.C., "Nutritional strategies to minimize exercise-induced immunosuppression in athletes," *Canadian Journal of Applied Physiology*, 26 (Suppl): S23–S35, 2001.

Ivy, J.L., "Dietary strategies to promote glycogen synthesis after exercise," *Canadian Journal of Applied Physiology*, 26 (Suppl): S236–S245, 2001.

Ivy, J.L., Katz, A.L., Cutler, C.L., et al., "Muscle glycogen synthesis after exercise: effect of time on carbohydrate ingestion," *Journal of Applied Physiology*, 64: 1480–1485, 1988.

Levenhagen, D.K., Carr, C., Carlson, M.G., et al., "Post exercise protein intake enhances whole-body and leg protein accretion in humans," *Medicine and Science in Sports and Exercise*, 34: 828–837, 2002.

Levenhagen, D.K., Gresham, J.D., Carlson, M.G., et al., "Post exercise nutrient intake timing in humans is critical to recovery of leg glucose and protein homeostasis," *American Journal Physiology*, 280: E982–E993, 2001.

Okano, G., Suzuki, M., Kojima, M., et al., "Effect of timing of meal intake after squat exercise training on bone formation in the rat hind limb," *Journal of Nutritional Science and Vitaminology*, 45: 543–552, 1999.

Suzuki, M., Doi, T., Lee, S.J., et al., "Effect of meal timing after resistance exercise on hind limb muscle mass and fat accumulation in trained rats," *Journal of Nutritional Science and Vitaminology*, 45: 401–409, 1999.

Van Loon, L.J.C., Saris, W.H.M., Verhagen, H., et al., "Plasma insulin responses following the ingestion of different amino acid and/or protein mixtures with carbohydrate," *American Journal of Clinical Nutrition*, 72: 96–105, 2000.

Zawadzki, K.M., Yaspelkis, B.B., III, and Ivy, J.L., "Carbohydrate-protein complex increases the rate of muscle glycogen storage after exercise," *Journal of Applied Physiology*, 72: 1854–1859, 1992.

Chapter 2: Muscle Energy Systems

Armstrong, R., "Biochemistry: energy liberation and use," IN: Sports Medicine and Physiology. Ed. Strauss, R. Philadelphia, W.B. Saunders, 1979.

Gollnick, P., "Metabolism of substances: energy substrate metabolism during exercise and as modified by training," *Federation Proceedings*, 44: 353–356, 1985.

Karlsson, J., "Lactate and phosphagen concentrations in working muscle of man," *Acta Physiologica Scandinavaca*, 358 (Suppl): 1–72, 1971.

McArdle, W.D., Katch, F.I., and Katch, V.L., Exercise Physiology, Energy, Nutrition, and Human Performance, (3rd edition), Philadelphia: Lea & Febiger, 1991.

Wilmore, J. H., and Costill, D.L., Training for Sport and Activity. The Physiological Basis of the Conditioning Process, (3rd edition), Dubuque, IA: Wm. C. Brown Publishers, 1988.

Chapter 3: The Influence of Hormones on Muscle Growth and Development

Baron, A.D., Steinberg, H., Brechtel, G., et al., "Skeletal muscle blood flow independently modulates insulin-mediated glucose uptake," *American Journal of Physiology*, 266: E248–E253, 1994.

Cumming, D.C., Wall, S.R., Galbraith, M.A., and Belcastro, A.N., "Reproductive hormonal responses to resistance exercise," *Medicine and Science in Sports and Exercise*, 19: 234–238, 1987.

Esmarck, B., Andersen, J.L., Olsen, S., et al., "Timing of post exercise protein intake is important for muscle hypertrophy with resistance training in elderly humans," *Journal of Physiology*, 535: 301–311, 2001.

Fahey, T. D., "Anabolic-androgenic steroids: mechanisms of action and effects on performance," IN: Encyclopedia of Sports Medicine and Science, T. D. Fahey (Editor). March 7, 1998.

Ferrando, A.A., Sheffield-Moore, M., Paddon-Jones, D., et al., "Differential anabolic effects of testosterone and amino acid feeding in older men," *Journal of Clinical Endocrinology and Metabolism*, 88: 358–362, 2003.

Ferrando, A.A., Tipton, K.D., Doyle, D., et al. "Testosterone injection stimulates net protein synthesis but not tissue amino acid transport," *American Journal of Physiology*, 275: E864–E871, 1998.

Gleeson, M., Lancaster, G.I., and Bishop, N.C., "Nutritional strategies to minimize exercise-induced immunosuppression in athletes," *Canadian Journal of Applied Physiology*, 26 (Suppl): S23–S35, 2001.

Guezennec, Y., Leger, L., Lhoste, F., Aymonod, M., and Pesquies, P.C., "Hormonal and metabolic responses to weightlifting training sessions," *International Journal of Sports Medicine*, 7: 100–105, 1986.

Kraemer, W.J., "Endocrine responses to resistance exercise," *Medicine and Science in Sports and Exercise*, 20: S152–S157, 1988.

Kraemer, W.J., Marchitelli, L., Gordon, S.E., et al., "Hormonal and growth factor responses to heavy resistance exercise protocols," *Journal of Applied Physiology*, 69: 1442–50, 1990.

Kraemer, W.J., Häkkinen, K., Newton, R.U., et al., "Effects of heavy-resistance training on hormonal response patterns in younger vs. older men," *Journal of Applied Physiology*, 87: 982–992, 1999.

Laakso, M., Edelman, S.V., Brechtel, G., et al., "Decreased effect of insulin to stimulate skeletal muscle blood flow in obese men: a novel mechanism for insulin release," *Journal of Clinical Investigation*. 85: 1844–1852, 1990.

Laakso, M., Edelman, S.V., Brechtel, G., et al., "Effects of epinephrine on insulin-mediated glucose uptake in whole body and leg muscle in humans: role of blood flow," *American Journal of Physiology*, 263: E199–E204, 1992.

Levenhagen, D.K., Gresham, J.D., Carlson, M.G., et al., "Post exercise nutrient intake timing in humans is critical to recovery of leg glucose and protein homeostasis," *American Journal of Endocrinology and Metabolism*, 280: E982–E993, 2001.

Lukaszewska, J., Biczowa, B., Bobilewicz, D., et al., "Effect of physical exercise on plasma cortisol and growth hormone levels in young weight lifters," *Endokrynology Polska*, 2: 149–158, 1976.

McMurray, R.G., Eubank, T.K., and Hackney, A.C., "Nocturnal hormonal responses to resistance exercise," *European Journal of Applied Physiology*, 72: 121–126, 1995.

Miller, W.J., Sherman, W.M., and Ivy, J.L., "Effect of strength training on glucose tolerance and post glucose insulin response," *Medicine and Science in Sports and Exercise*, 16: 539–543, 1984.

O'Connor, P.M., Bush, J.A., Surywan, A., et al., "Insulin and amino acids independently stimulate skeletal muscle protein synthesis in neonatal pigs," *American Journal of Physiology*, 284: E110–E119, 2003.

O'Connor, P.M.J., Kimball S.R., Suryawan, A., et al., "Regulation of translation initiation by insulin and amino acids in skeletal muscle of neonatal pigs," *American Journal of Physiology*, 285: E40–E53, 2003.

Van Loon, L.J., Kruijshoop, M., Verhagen, H., et al., "Ingestion of protein hydrolysate and amino acid-carbohydrate mixtures increases post exercise plasma insulin responses in men, *Journal of Nutrition*, 130: 2508–2513, 2000.

Van Loon, L.J., Saris, W.H.M., Kruijshoop, M., et al., "Maximizing post exercise muscle glycogen synthesis: carbohydrate supplementation and the application of amino acid or protein hydrolysate mixtures," *American Journal of Clinical Nutrition*, 72: 106–111, 2000.

Van Loon, L.J.C., Saris, W.H.M., Verhagen, H., et al., "Plasma insulin responses following the ingestion of different amino acid and/or protein mixtures with carbohydrate," *American Journal of Clinical Nutrition*, 72: 96–105, 2000.

Zawadzki, K.M., Yaspelkis, B.B., III, and Ivy, J.L., "Carbohydrate-protein complex increases the rate of muscle glycogen storage after exercise," *Journal of Applied Physiology*, 72: 1854–1859, 1992.

Chapter 4: NTS Energy Phase

Bigard, A.X., Sanchez, H., Claveyrolas, G., et al., "Effects of dehydration and rehydration on EMG changes during fatiguing contractions," *International Journal of Sports Medicine*, 8: 281–285, 1987.

Bishop, N.C., Blannin, A.K., Rand, L., et al., "Effects of carbohydrate and fluid intake on the blood leukocyte responses to prolonged cycling," *International Journal of Sport Medicine*, 17: 26–27, 1999.

Bishop, N.C., Blannin, A.K., Rand, L., et al., "The effects of carbohydrate supplementation on neutrophil degranulation responses to prolonged cycling," *International Journal of Sport Medicine*, 21(Suppl 1): S73, 2000.

Bishop, N.C., Blannin, A.K., Walsh, N.P., et al., "Carbohydrate beverage ingestion and neutrophil degranulation responses following cycling to fatigue at 75% VO_2 max," *International Journal of Sport Medicine*, 22: 226–231, 2001.

Gleeson, M., Blannin, A.K., Walsh, N.P., et al., "Effect of low and high carbohydrate diets on the plasma glutamine and circulating leukocyte responses to exercise," *International Journal of Sport Medicine*, 8: 49–59, 1998.

Haff, G.G., Koch, A.J., Potteiger, J.A., et al., "Carbohydrate supplementation attenuates muscle glycogen loss during acute bouts of resistance exercise," *International Journal of Sport Nutrition and Exercise Metabolism*, 10: 326–339, 2000.

Haff, G.G., Lehmkuhl, M.J., McCoy, L.B., et al., "Carbohydrate supplementation and resistance training," *Journal of Strength and Conditioning Research*, 17: 187–196, 2003.

Haff, G.G., Schroeder, C.A., Koch, A.J., et al., "The effects of supplemental carbohydrate ingestion on intermittent isokinetic leg exercise," *Journal of Sports Medicine and Physical Fitness*. 41: 216–222, 2001.

Hargreaves, M., Costill, D.L., Coggan, A.R., et al., "Effect of carbohydrate feedings on muscle glycogen utilization and exercise performance," *Medicine and Science in Sport and Exercise*, 16: 219–225, 1984.

Hurst, T.L., Bailey, D.M., Powell, J.R., et al., "Immune function changes in downhill running subjects following ascorbic acid supplementation," *Medicine and Science in Sports and Exercise*, 33(Suppl 5): S35, 2001.

Ivy, J.L., "Optimization of glycogen stores," IN: Encyclopaedia of Sports Medicine: Nutrition in Sports. (Ed.) S. Knuttgen. Blackwell Science Ltd. Oxford, UK, 2000, pg. 97–111.

Ivy, J.L., Res, P.T., Sprague, R.C., et al., "Effect of carbohydrate-protein supplement on endurance performance during exercise of varying intensity," *International Journal of Sport Nutrition and Exercise Metabolism*, 13: 388–401, 2003.

Kalliokoski, K.K., Kemppainen, J., Larmola, K., et al., "Muscle blood flow and flow heterogeneity during exercise studied with positron emission tomography in humans," *European Journal of Applied Physiology*, 83: 395–401, 2000.

MacLean, D.A., Graham, T.E. and Saltin, B., "Branched-chain amino acids augment ammonia metabolism while attenuating protein breakdown during exercise," *American Journal of Physiology*, 267: E1010–1022, 1994.

Nehlsen-Cannarella, S.L., Fagoaga, O.R., Neiman, D.C., et al., "Carbohydrate and the cytokine response to 2.5 hours of running," *Journal of Applied Physiology*, 82: 1662–1667, 1997.

Nieman, D.C., "Nutrition, exercise, and immune system function," IN: Clinicals in Sports Medicine, Nutritional Aspects of Exercise. Eds. Wheeler, K.B. and Lombardo, J.A. Vol. 18, 1999, p 537–538.

Nieman, D.C., Johansen, L.M., Lee, J.W., et al., "Infectious episodes in runners before and after the Los Angeles Marathon," *Journal of Sports Medicine and Physical Fitness*, 30: 316–328, 1990.

Peters, E.M., Goetzsche, J.M., Grobbelaar, B., et al., "Vitamin C supplementation reduced the incidence of post-race symptoms of upper respiratory tract infection in ultra marathon runners," *American Journal of Clinical Nutrition*, 57: 170–174, 1993.

Ploutz-Snyder, L.L., Convertino, V.A., and Dudley, G.A., "Resistance exercise-induced fluid shifts: change in active muscle size and plasma volume," *American Journal of Physiology*, 269: R536–R543, 1995.

Potteiger, J.A., Chan, M.A., Haff, G.G., et al., "Training status influences T-cell responses in women following acute resistance exercise," *Journal Strength and Conditioning Research*, 15: 185–191, 2001.

Robergs, R.A., Pearson, D.R., and Costill, D.L., "Muscle glycogenolysis during differing intensities of weight-resistance exercise," *Journal of Applied Physiology*, 70: 1700–1706, 1991.

Rokitzki, L., Logeman, E., Sagredos, A.N., et al., "Lipid peroxidation and antioxidant vitamins under extreme endurance stress," *Acta Physiologica Scandinavacia*, 151: 149–158, 1994.

Rokitzki, L., Logemann, E., Huber, G., et al., "alpha-Tocopherol supplementation in racing cyclists during extreme endurance training," *International Journal of Sport Nutrition*, 4: 253–264, 1994.

Schoffstall, J.E., Branch, J.D., Leutholtz, B.C., et al., "Effects of dehydration and rehydration on the one-repetition maximum branch press of weight-trained males," *Medicine and Science in Sports and Exercise*, 33: 1694–1700, 2001.

Tesch, P.A., Colliander, E.B., and Kaiser P., "Muscle metabolism during intense, heavy-resistance exercise," *European Journal of Physiology and Occupational Physiology,* 55: 362–366, 1986.

Viitasalo, J.T., Kyrolainen, H., Bosco, C., and Alen, M., "Effects of rapid weight reduction on force production and vertical jumping heights," *International Journal of Sports Medicine,* 8: 281–285, 1987.

Yaspelkis, B.B., Patterson, J.G., Anderla, P.A., et al., "Carbohydrate supplementation spares muscle glycogen during variable-intensity exercise," *Journal of Applied Physiology,* 75: 1477–1485, 1993.

Chapter 5: NTS Anabolic Phase

Andersen, J.L., Schjerling, P., Andersen, L.L., and Dela, F., "Resistance training and insulin action in humans: effects of de-training," *Journal of Physiology,* 551: 1049–1058, 2003.

Anthony, J.C., Anthony, T.G., and Layman, D.K., "Leucine supplementation enhances skeletal muscle recovery in rats following exercise," *Journal of Nutrition,* 129: 1102–1106, 1999.

Biolo, G., Tipton, K.D., Klein, S., et al., "An abundant supply of amino acids enhances the metabolic effect of exercise on muscle protein," *American Journal of Physiology,* 273: E122–E119, 1997.

Boirie, Y., Dangin, M., Gachon, P., et al., "Slow and fast dietary proteins differently modulate postprandial protein accretion," *Proceedings of the National Academy of Sciences USA,* 94: 14930–12935, 1997.

Blomstrand, E., and Saltin B., "BCAA intake affects protein metabolism in muscle after but not during exercise in human," *American Journal of Physiology,* 28: E365–E374, 2001.

Cardillo, C., Kilcoyne, C.M., Nambi, S.S., et al., "Vasodilator response to systemic but not local hyperinsulemia in the human forearm," *Hypertension,* 34: E12–E13, 1999.

Chandler, R.M., Byrne, H.K., Patterson, J.G., and Ivy, J.L., "Dietary supplements affect the anabolic hormones after high resistance exercise," *Journal of Applied Physiology,* 76: 839–845, 1994.

Clark, M.W., Wallis, M.D., Barrett, E.J., et al., "Blood flow and muscle metabolism: a focus on insulin action," *American Journal of Physiology,* 284: E241–E258, 2003.

Dangin, M., Boirie, Y., Garcia-Rodenas, C., et al., "The digestion rate of protein is an independent regulating factor of postprandial protein retention," *American Journal of Physiology,* 280: E340–348, 2001.

Esmarck, B., Andersen, J.L., Olsen, S., et al., "Timing of postexercise protein intake is important for muscle hypertrophy with resistance training in elderly humans," *Journal of Physiology,* 535: 301–311, 2001.

Gautsch, T.A., Anthony, J.C., Kimball, S.R., et al., "Availability of eIF4E regulates skeletal muscle protein synthesis during recovery from exercise," *American Journal of Physiology,* 274: C406–C414, 1998.

Ivy, J.L., "Dietary strategies to promote glycogen synthesis after exercise," *Canadian Journal of Applied Physiology,* 26 (Suppl): S236–S245, 2001.

Ivy, J.L., Katz, A.L., Cutler, C.L., et al., "Muscle glycogen synthesis after exercise: effect of time on carbohydrate ingestion," *Journal of Applied Physiology*, 64: 1480–1485, 1988.

Ivy, J.L., Goforth, H.W., Jr., Damon, B.M., et al., "Early post exercise muscle glycogen recovery is enhanced with a carbohydrate-protein supplement," *Journal of Applied Physiology*, 93: 1337–1344, 2002.

Jun, T., and Wennmalm, A., "NO-dependent and –independent elevation of plasma levels of insulin and glucose in rats by L-arginine," *British Journal of Pharmacology*, 113: 345–348, 1994.

King, N.A., Burley, V.J., and Blundell, J.E., "Exercise-induced suppression of appetite: effects on food intake and implications for energy balance," *European Journal of Clinical Nutrition*, 48: 715–24, 1994.

Laakso, M., Edelman, S.V., Brechtel, G., and Baron, A.D., "Decreased effect of insulin to stimulate skeletal muscle blood flow in obese man: a novel mechanism for insulin resistance," *Journal of Clinical Investigation*, 85: 1844–1852, 1990.

Levenhagen, D.K., Carr, C., Carlson, M.G., et al., "Postexercise protein intake enhances whole-body and leg protein accretion in humans," *Medicine and Science in Sports and Exercise*, 34: 828–837, 2002.

Levenhagen, D.K., Gresham, J.D., Carlson, M.G., et al., "Postexercise nutrient intake timing in humans is critical to recovery of leg glucose and protein homeostasis," *American Journal of Physiology*, 280: E982–E993, 2001.

Okamura, K., Doi, T., Hamada, K., et al., "Effect of amino acid and glucose administration during postexercise recovery on protein kinetics in dogs," *American Journal of Physiology*," 272: E1023–E1030, 1997.

Okano, G., Suzuki, M., Kojima, M., et al., "Effect of timing of meal intake after squat exercise training on bone formation in the rat hind limb," *Journal of Nutritional Science and Vitaminology*, 45: 543–552, 1999.

Ready, S.L., Seifert, J., Burke, E., "Effect of two sports drinks on muscle tissue stress and performance," *Medicine and Science in Sports and Exercise*, 31(5): S119, 1999.

Roy, B.D., Fowles, J.R., Hill, R., et al., "Macronutrient intake and whole body protein metabolism following resistance exercise," *Medicine and Science in Sports and Exercise*, 32: 1412–1418, 2000.

Roy, B.D., Tarnopolsky, M.A., MacDougall J.D., et al., "Effect of glucose supplement timing on protein metabolism after resistance training," *Journal of Applied Physiology*, 82: 1882–1888, 1997.

Spiller, G.A., Jensen, C.D., Pattison, T.S., et al., "Effect of protein dose on serum glucose and insulin response to sugars," *American Journal of Clinical Nutrition*, 46: 474–481, 1987.

Suzuki, M., Doi, T., Lee, S.J., et al., "Effect of meal timing after resistance exercise on hind limb muscle mass and fat accumulation in trained rats," *Journal of Nutritional Science and Vitaminology*, 45: 401–409, 1999.

Tarnopolsky, M.A., Bosman, M., MacDonald, J.R., et al., "Post exercise protein-carbohydrate and carbohydrate supplements increase muscle glycogen in men and women," *Journal of Applied Physiology*, 83: 1877–1883, 1997.

Utrainen, T., Mäkimatilla, S., Virkamäki, A., et al., "Physical fitness and endothelial function (nitric oxide synthesis) are independent determinants of insulin-stimulated blood flow in normal subjects," *Journal of Endocrinology and Metabolism*, 81: 4258–4263, 1996.

van der Schoor, P., van Hall, G., Saris, W.H.M., et al., "Ingestion of protein hydrolysate prevents the post-exercise reduction in plasma glutamate," *International Journal of Sports Medicine*, 18: S115, 1997.

van Loon, L.J.C., Saris, W.H.M., Verhagen, H., et al., "Plasma insulin responses following the ingestion of different amino acid and/or protein mixtures with carbohydrate," *American Journal of Clinical Nutrition*, 72: 96–105, 2000.

Williams, M., Ivy, J., Raven, P., "Effects of recovery drinks after prolonged glycogen-depletion exercise," *Medicine and Science in Sports and Exercise*, 31(5):S124, 1999.

Williams, M.B., Raven, P.B., Donovan L.F., et al., "Effects of recovery beverage on glycogen restoration and endurance exercise performance," *Journal of Strength and Conditioning Research*, 17: 12–19, 2003.

Yki-Jarvinen, H., "Insulin resistance and endothelial dysfunction," *Best Practice and Research Clinical Endocrinology and Metabolism*, 17: 411–430, 2003.

Zawadzki, K.M., Yaspelkis, B.B., III, and Ivy, J.L., "Carbohydrate-protein complex increases the rate of muscle glycogen storage after exercise," *Journal of Applied Physiology*, 72: 1854–1859, 1992.

Chapter 6: NTS Growth Phase

Anthony, J.C., Anthony, T.G., and Layman, D.K., "Leucine supplementation enhances skeletal muscle recovery in rats following exercise," *Journal of Nutrition*, 129: 1102–1106, 1999.

Apple, F.S., Rogers, M.A., Sherman, W.M., et al., "Comparison of serum creatine kinase and creatine kinase MB activities post marathon race versus post myocardial infarction," *Clinica Chimica Acta.* 138: 111–118, 1984.

Biolo, G., Tipton, K.D., Klein, S., et al., "An abundant supply of amino acids enhances the metabolic effect of exercise on muscle protein," *American Journal of Physiology*, 273: E122–E119, 1997.

Blom, P.C.S., Høstmark, A.T., Vaage, O., et al., "Effect of different post-exercise sugar diets on the rate of muscle glycogen synthesis," *Medicine and Science in Sports and Exercise*, 19: 491–496, 1987.

Boirie, Y., Dangin, M., Gachon, P., et al., "Slow and fast dietary proteins differently modulate postprandial protein accretion," *Proceedings of the National Academy of Sciences, USA*, 94: 14930–12935, 1997.

Borsheim, E., Tipton, K.D., Wolf, S.E., and Wolfe, R.R., "Essential amino acids and muscle protein recovery from resistance exercise," *American Journal of Physiology*, 283: E648–E657, 2002.

Chittenden, R.H., The Nutrition of Man. Heinemann, London, 1907.

Evans, W.J., "Protein nutrition and resistance exercise," *Canadian Journal of Applied Physiology*, 26 (Suppl): S141–S152, 2001.

Fielding, R.A., and Parkington, J., "What are the dietary protein requirements of physically active individuals? New evidence on the effects of exercise on protein utilization during postexercise recovery," *Nutrition and Clinical Care*, 5: 191–196, 2002.

Fern, E.B., Bielinski, R.N., and Schutz, Y., "Effects of exaggerated amino acid and protein supply in man," *Experientia*, 47: 168–172, 1991.

Forslund, A.H., El-Khoury, A.E., Olsson, R.M., et al., "Effect of protein intake and physical activity on 24-h pattern and rate of macronutrient utilization," *American Journal or Physiology*, 276: E964–E976, 1999.

Forslund, A.H., Habraeus, L., Olsson, R.M., et al., "The 24-h whole body leucine and urea kinetics at normal and high protein intake with exercise in healthy adults," *American Journal of Physiology*, 275: E310–E320, 1998.

Forslund, A.H., Habraeus, L., Van Beurden, H., et al., "Inverse relationship between protein intake and plasma free amino acids in healthy men at physical exercise," *American Journal of Physiology*, 278: E857–E867, 2000.

Gater, D.R., Gater, D.A., Uribe, J.M., et al., "Impact of nutritional supplements and resistance training on body composition, strength and insulin-like growth factor-1," *Journal of Applied Sports Science Research*, 6: 66–76, 1992.

Gautsch, T.A., Anthony, J.C., Kimball, S.R., et al., "Availability of eIF4E regulates skeletal muscle protein synthesis during recovery from exercise," *American Journal of Physiology*, 274: C406–C414, 1998.

Haff, G.G., Koch, A.J, Potteiger, J.A., et al., "Carbohydrate supplementation attenuates muscle glycogen loss during acute bouts of resistance exercise," *International Journal of Sport Nutrition and Exercise Metabolism*, 10: 326–339, 2000.

Haff, G.G., Lehmkuhl, M.J., McCoy, L.B., et al., "Carbohydrate supplementation and resistance training," *Journal of Strength and Conditioning Research*, 17: 187–196, 2003.

Hegsted, M., et al., "Urinary calcium and calcium balance in young men as affected by level of protein and phosphorous intake," *Journal of Nutrition*, 111: 553–562, 1991.

Ivy, J.L., Katz, A.L., Cutler, C.L., et al., "Muscle glycogen synthesis after exercise: effect of time of carbohydrate ingestion," *Journal of Applied Physiology*, 64: 1480–1485, 1988.

Ivy, J.L., Lee, M.C., Brozinick, J.T., et al., "Muscle glycogen storage after different amounts of carbohydrate ingestion," *Journal of Applied Physiology*, 65: 2018–2023, 1988.

Lemon, P.W., Dolny, D.G., Yarasheski, K.E., "Moderate physical activity can increase dietary protein needs," *Canadian Journal of Applied Physiology*, 22: 494–503, 1997.

Levenhagen, D.K., Gresham, J.D., Carlson, M.G., et al., "Post-exercise nutrient intake timing in humans is critical to recovery of leg glucose and protein homeostasis," *American Journal of Physiology*, 280: E982–E993, 2001.

Miller, S.L., Tipton, K.D., Chinkes, D.L., et al., "Independent and combined effects of amino acids and glucose after resistance exercise," *Medicine and Science in Sports and Exercise*, 35: 449–455, 2003.

National Academy of Sciences National Research Council, Recommended Dietary Allowances, (9th edition), Washington, D.C.: National Academy Press, 1989.

Oddoye, E.A., Margen, S., "Nitrogen balance studies in humans: long-term effect of high nitrogen intake on nitrogen accretion," *Journal of Nutrition*, 109: 363–377, 1979.

Phillips, S.M., Tipton, K.D., Aarsland, S.E., et al., "Mixed muscle protein synthesis and breakdown after resistance exercise in humans," *American Journal of Physiology*, 273: E99–E107, 1997.

Poortmans, J.R., and Dellalieux, O., "Do regular high protein diets have potential health risks on kidney function in athletes?" *International Journal of Sport Nutrition and Exercise Metabolism*, 10: 28–38, 2000.

Rasmussen, B.B., Tipton, K.D., Miller, S.L., et al., "An oral essential amino acid-carbohydrate supplement enhances muscle protein anabolism after resistance exercise," *Journal of Applied Physiology*, 88: 386–392, 2000.

Sterck, J.G., Ritskes-Hoitinga, J., and Beynen, A.C., "Inhibitory effect of high protein intake on nephrocalcinogenesis in female rats," *British Journal of Nutrition*, 67: 223–233, 1992.

Suzuki, M., Doi, T., Lee, S.J., et al., "Effect of meal timing after resistance exercise on hind-limb muscle mass and fat accumulation in trained rats," *Journal of Nutritional Science and Vitaminology*, 45: 401–409, 1999.

Tarnopolsky, M.A., "Protein and physical performance," *Current Opinions on Clinical Nutrition and Metabolic Care*, 2: 533–537, 1999.

Tarnopolsky, M.A., Atkinson, S.A., MacDougall, J.D., et al., "Whole body leucine metabolism during and after resistance exercise in fed humans," *Medicine and Science in Sports and Exercise*, 23: 326–333, 1991.

Tarnopolsky, M.A., MacDougall, J.D., Atkinson, S.A., "Influence of protein intake and training status on nitrogen balance and lean body mass," *Journal of Applied Physiology*, 64: 187–193, 1988.

Wolfe, R.R., "Effects of amino acid intake on anabolic processes," *Canadian Journal of Applied Physiology*, 26: S220–S227, 2001.

Chapter 7: Making Nutrient Timing Work for You

Ballor, D.L., Becque, M.D., Katch, V.L., "Metabolic responses during hydraulic resistance exercise," *Medicine and Science in Sports Exercise*, 19: 363–367, 1987.

Beckham, S.G., and Earnest, C.P., "Metabolic cost of free weight circuit weight training," *Journal of Sports Medicine and Physical Fitness*, 40: 118–25, 2000.

Ivy, J.L., "Dietary strategies to promote glycogen synthesis after exercise," *Canadian Journal of Applied Physiology*, 26 (Suppl): S236–S245, 2001.

Ivy, J.L., Goforth, H.W., Jr., Damon, B.M., et al., "Early postexercise muscle glycogen recovery is enhanced with a carbohydrate-protein supplement," *Journal of Applied Physiology*, 93: 1337–1344, 2002.

Ivy, J.L., Katz, A.L., Cutler, C.L., et al., "Muscle glycogen synthesis after exercise: effect of time on carbohydrate ingestion," *Journal of Applied Physiology*, 64: 1480–1485, 1988.

Lemon, P.W., Dolny, D.G., Yarasheski, K.E., "Moderate physical activity can increase dietary protein needs," *Canadian Journal of Applied Physiology*, 22: 494–503, 1997.

Levenhagen, D.K., Gresham, J.D., Carlson, M.G., et al., "Postexercise nutrient intake timing in humans is critical to recovery of leg glucose and protein homeostasis," *American Journal Physiology*, 280: E982–E993, 2001.

Miller, S.L., Tipton, K.D., Chinkes, D.L, et al., "Independent and combined effects of amino acids and glucose after resistance exercise," *Medicine and Science in Sports and Exercise*, 35: 449–455, 2003.

National Academy of Sciences National Research Council, Recommended Dietary Allowances, (9th edition), Washington, D.C.: National Academy Press, 1989.

Wilmore, J.H., Parr, R.B., Ward, P., et al., "Energy cost of circuit weight training," *Medicine and Science in Sports*, 10: 75–78, 1978.

Wolfe, R.R., "Effects of amino acid intake on anabolic processes," *Canadian Journal of Applied Physiology*, 26: S220–S227, 2001.

CHAPTER 7: LIQUID NUTRITION VERSUS FOOD (INSET)

Dangin, M., Boirie, Y., Garcia-Rodenas, C., Gachon, P., Fauquant, J., Callier, P., Ballevre, O., Beaufrere, B., "The digestion rate of protein is an independent regulating factor of postprandial protein retention," *American Journal of Physiology*, 280: E340–E348, 2001.

King, N.A., Burley, V.J., Blundell, J.E., "Exercise-induced suppression of appetite: effects on food intake and implications for energy balance," *European Journal of Clinical Nutrition*, 48: 715–724, 1994.

Levenhagen, D.K., Gresham, J.D., Carlson, M.G., Maron, D.J., Borel, M.J., Flakoll, P.J., "Postexercise nutrient intake timing in humans is critical to recovery of leg glucose and protein homeostasis," *American Journal of Physiology*, 280: E982–E993, 2001.

Chapter 8: The NTS Program

American Diabetes Association, American Dietetic Association, Exchange Lists for Meal Planning, 2003.

Ivy, J.L., "Dietary strategies to promote glycogen synthesis after exercise," *Canadian Journal of Applied Physiology*, 26 (Suppl): S236–245, 2001.

Kleiner, S.M., Greenwood-Robinson, M., Power Eating, (2nd edition), Human Kinetics Publishers, Champaign, IL, 2001.

Kleiner, S.M., "Water: an essential but overlooked nutrient," *Journal of the American Dietetic Association*, 99: 200–206, 1999.

Zemel, M.B., "Regulation of adiposity and obesity risk by dietary calcium: mechanisms and implications," *Journal of the American College of Nutritionists*, 21(2): 146S–151S, 2002.

CHAPTER 8: ARE HIGH-PROTEIN DIETS AND PROTEIN SUPPLEMENTS DANGEROUS? (INSET)

Hegsted, M., et al., "Urinary calcium and calcium balance in young men as affected by level of protein and phosphorus intake," *Journal of Nutrition*, 111: 553–562, 1991.

National Academy of Sciences National Research Council. *Recommended dietary allowances* (9th ed). Washington, D.C.; National Academy Press, 1989.

Poortmans, J.R., and Dellalieux, O., "Do regular high protein diets have potential health risks on kidney function in athletes?" *International Journal of Sport Nutrition and Exercise Metabolism*, 10: 28–38, 2000.

Sterck, et al., "Inhibitory effect of high protein intake on nephrocalcinogenesis in female rats," *British Journal of Nutrition*, 67: 223–233, 1992.

Chapter 9: Nutrient Activators and Sports Supplements

Anthony, J.C., Anthony, T.G., and Layman, D.K., "Leucine supplementation enhances skeletal muscle recovery in rats following exercise," *Journal of Nutrition*, 129: 1102–1106, 1999.

Bell, D.G., and McLellan, T.M., "Exercise endurance 1, 3, and 6 h after caffeine ingestion in caffeine users and nonusers," *Journal of Applied Physiology*, 93: 1227–1234, 2002.

Biolo, G., Tipton, K.D., Klein, S., et al., "An abundant supply of amino acids enhances the metabolic effect of exercise on muscle protein," *American Journal of Physiology*, 273: E122–E119, 1997.

Bishop, N.C., Blannin, A.K., Walsh, N.P., et al., "Nutritional aspects of immunosuppression in athletes," *Sport Medicine*, 28: 151–176, 1999.

Blomstrand, E., Hassmen, P., Ekblom, B., and Newsholme, E.A., "Administration of branched chain amino acids during sustained exercise: effects on performance and on plasma concentration of some amino acids," *European Journal of Applied Physiology and Occupational Physiology*, 63: 83–88, 1991.

Bowtell, J.L., Gelly, K., Jackman, M.L., et al., "Effect of oral glutamine on whole body carbohydrate storage during recovery from exhaustive exercise," *Journal of Applied Physiology*, 86: 1770–1777, 1999.

Bruce, C.R., Anderson, M.E., Fraser, S.F., et al., "Enhancement of 2000-m rowing performance after caffeine ingestion," *Medicine and Science in Sports and Exercise*, 32: 1958–1963, 2000.

Castell, L.M., and Newsholme, E.A., "The effects of oral glutamine supplementation on athletes after prolonged, exhaustive exercise," *Nutrition*, 13: 738–742, 1997.

Coombes, J.S., and McNaughton, L.R., "Effects of branched-chain amino acid supplementation on serum creatine kinase and lactate dehydrogenase after prolonged exercise," *Journal of Sports Medicine and Physical Fitness,* 40: 240–246, 2000.

Costill, D.L., Dalsky, G.P., and Fink, W.J., "Effects of caffeine ingestion on metabolism and exercise performance," *Medicine and Science in Sports,* 10: 155–158, 1978.

Davis, J.M., Zhao, Z., Stock, H.S., et al., "Central nervous system effects of caffeine and adenosine on fatigue," *American Journal of Physiology,* 284: R399–R404, 2003.

Green, A.L., et al., "Carbohydrate feeding augments creatine retention during creatine feeding in humans," *American Journal of Physiology,* 271: E821–E826, 1996.

Ivy, J.L., "Effect of pyruvate and dihydroxyacetone supplementation on metabolism and aerobic endurance capacity," *Medicine and Science in Sports and Exercise,* 30: 837–843, 1998.

Ivy, J.L., Costill, D.L., Fink, W.J., and Lower, R.W., "Influence of caffeine and carbohydrate feedings on endurance performance," *Medicine and Science in Sports,* 11: 6–11, 1979.

Juhn, M., "Popular sports supplements and ergogenic aids," *Sports Medicine,* 33: 921–939, 2003.

Kingsbury, K.J., Kay, L., and Hjelm, M., "Contrasting plasma free amino acid patterns in elite athletes: association with fatigue and infection," *British Journal of Sports Medicine,* 32: 25–32, 1998.

Kreider, R.B., Ferreira, M., Wilson, M., et al., "Effects of creatine supplementation on body composition, strength, and sprint performance," *Medicine and Science in Sports and Exercise,* 30: 73–82, 1998.

Kraemer, W.J., Volek, J.S., French, D.N., et al., "The effects of L-carnitine L-tartrate supplementation on hormonal responses to resistance exercise and recovery," *Journal of Strength Conditioning Research,* 17(3): 455–462, 2003.

Laurent, D., Schneider, K.E., Prusaczyk, W.K., et al., "Effects of caffeine on muscle glycogen utilization and the neuroendocrine axis during exercise," *Journal of Clinical Endocrinology and Metabolism,* 85: 2170–175, 2000.

MacLennan, P.A., Smith, K., Weryk, B., et al., "Inhibition of protein breakdown by glutamine in perfused rat skeletal muscle," *FEBS Letters,* 237: 133–136, 1988.

MacLennan, P.A., Brown, R.A., and Rennie, M.J., "A positive relationship between protein synthetic rate and intracellular glutamine concentration in perfused rat skeletal muscle," *FEBS Letters,* 215: 187–191, 1987.

Maiorana, A., O'Driscoll, G., Taylor, R., and Green, D., "Exercise and the nitric oxide vasodilator system," *Sports Medicine,* 33: 1013–35, 2003.

Miller, S.L., Tipton, K.D., Chinkes, D.L., et al., "Independent and combined effects of amino acids and glucose after resistance exercise," *Medicine and Science in Sports and Exercise,* 35: 449–455, 2003.

Nissen, S.L., Sharp, R.L., "Effect of dietary supplements on lean mass and strength gains with resistance exercise: a meta-analysis," *Journal of Applied Physiology,* 94: 651–659, 2003.

Nissen, S., Sharp, R., Ray, M., et al., "Effect of leucine metabolite beta-hydroxy-beta-methylbutyrate on muscle metabolism during resistance-exercise training," *Journal of Applied Physiology*, 81: 2095–2104, 1996.

Peters, E.M., Anderson, R., and Theron, A.J., "Attenuation of increase in circulating cortisol and enhancement of the acute phase protein response in vitamin C-supplemented ultramarathoners," *International Journal of Sports Medicine*, 22: 120–126, 2001.

Ransone, J., Neighbors, K., Lefavi, R., Chromiak, J., "The effect of beta-hydroxy beta-methylbutyrate on muscular strength and body composition in collegiate football players," *Journal of Strength Conditioning Research*, 17: 34–39, 2003.

Rennie, M., Ahmed, A., Khogali, S.E., et al., "Glutamine metabolism and transport in skeletal muscle and heart and their clinical relevance," *Journal of Nutrition*, 126: 1142S–1149S, 1996.

Sacheck, J.M., and Blumberg, J.B., "Role of vitamin E and oxidative stress in exercise," *Nutrition*, 17: 809–14, 2001.

Sacheck, J.M., Milbury, P.E., Cannon, J.G., et al., "Effect of vitamin E and eccentric exercise on selected biomarkers of oxidative stress in young and elderly men," *Free Radical Biological Medicine*, 34: 1575–88, 2003.

Stehle, P., Zander, J., Mertes, N., et al., "Effect of parenteral glutamine peptide supplements on muscle glutamine loss and nitrogen balance after major surgery," *Lancet*, 1: 231–233, 1989.

Stone, M.H., Sanborn, K., Smith, L.L., et al., "Effects of in-season (5 weeks) creatine and pyruvate supplementation on anaerobic performance and body composition in American football players," *International Journal of Sport Nutrition*, 9: 146–65, 1999.

Stout, J., Eckerson, J., Noonan, D., et al., "Effects of 8 weeks of creatine supplementation on exercise performance and fat-free weight in football players during training," *Nutrition Research*, 19(2): 217–225, 1999.

Terpstra, A.H., Javadi, M., Beynen, A.C., et al., "Dietary conjugated linoleic acids as free fatty acids and triacylglycerols similarly affect body composition and energy balance in mice," *Journal of Nutrition*, 133: 3181–3186, 2003.

Thompson, D., Williams, C., McGregor, S.J., et al., "Prolonged vitamin C supplementation and recovery from demanding exercise," *International Journal of Sport Nutrition and Exercise Metabolism*, 11: 466–481, 2001.

Vandenberghe, K., Goris, M., Van Hecke, P., et al., "Long-term creatine intake is beneficial to muscle performance during resistance training," *Journal of Applied Physiology*, 83: 2055–2063, 1997.

Varnier, M., Leese, G.P., Thompson, J., et al., "Stimulatory effect of glutamine on glycogen accumulation in human skeletal muscle," *American Journal of Physiology*, 269: E309–E315, 1995.

Vom Dahl, S., and Haussinger, D., "Nutritional state and the swelling-induced inhibition of proteolysis in perfused rat liver," *Journal of Nutrition*, 126: 395–402, 1996.

Chapter 10: The Right Ingredients: Macronutrients

Campbell, W.W., Barton, M.L., Jr., Cyr-Campbell, D., et al., "Effects of an omnivorous diet compared with a lactoovovegetarian diet on resistance-training-induced changes in body composition and skeletal muscle in older men," *American Journal of Clinical Nutrition*, 79: 1032–1039, 1999.

Campbell, W.W., Crim, M.C., Young, V.R., et al., "Effects of resistance training and dietary protein intake on protein metabolism in older adults," *American Journal of Physiology*, 268: E1143–E1153, 1995.

Campbell, W.W., Crim, M.C., Young, V.R., and Evans, W.J., "Increased energy requirements and changes in body composition with resistance training in older adults," *American Journal of Clinical Nutrition*, 60: 167–175, 1995.

Fry, A.C., Kraemer, W.J., and Ramsey, L.T., "Pituitary-adrenal-gonadal responses to high-intensity resistance exercise overtraining," *Journal of Applied Physiology*, 85: 2352–2359, 1998.

Wilmore, J.H., and Costill, D.L., *Training for Sport and Activity: The Physiological Basis of the Conditioning Process*, (3rd edition), Dubuque, IA: Wm. C. Brown Publishers, 1988.

CHAPTER 10: VEGETARIAN MUSCLE BUILDING (INSET)

Campbell, W.W., et al., "Effects of an Omnivorous Diet Compared with a Lacto-ovovegetarian Diet on Resistance-Training-Induced Changes in Body Composition and Skeletal Muscle in Older Men," *American Journal of Clinical Nutrition*, 79: 1032–1039, 1999.

Campbell, W.W., et al., "Effects of resistance training and dietary protein intake on protein metabolism in older adults," *American Journal of Physiology*, 268: E1143–E1153, 1995.

Campbell, W.W., et al., "Increased energy requirements and changes in body composition with resistance training in older adults," *American Journal of Clinical Nutrition*, 60: 167–175, 1995.

CHAPTER 10: OVERTRAINING AND NUTRITION (INSET)

Fry, A.C., et al., "Pituitary-adrenal-gonadal responses to high-intensity resistance exercise overtraining," *Journal of Applied Physiology*, 85: 2352–2359, 1998.

Wilmore, J. H., and Costill, D.L., *Training for Sport and Activity: The Physiological Basis of the Conditioning Process* (3rd edition), Dubuque, IA: Wm. C. Brown Publishers, 1988.

Chapter 11: The Right Ingredients: Micronutrients

Chen, J., "Vitamins: effects of exercise," IN: Nutrition in Sports, Ed. Maughan, J. Oxford, England: Blackwell Science, 2000, pp. 281–291.

Clarkson, P.M., "Trace minerals," IN: Nutrition in Sports, Ed. Maughan, J. Oxford, England: Blackwell Science, 2000, 339–355.

Manore, M.M., "Effect of physical activity on thiamine, riboflavin, and vitamin B-6 requirements," *American Journal of Clinical Nutrition*, 72(2 Suppl): 598S–606S, 2000.

Maughan, R.J., "Role of micronutrients in sport and physical activity," *British Medical Bulletin*, 55: 683–690, 1999.

Peters, E.M., Goetzsche, J.M., Grobbelaar, B., et al., "Vitamin C supplementation reduces the incidence of post-race symptoms of upper respiratory tract in ultramarathon runner," *American Journal of Clinical Nutrition*, 57: 170–174, 1993.

Sacheck, J.M., Milbury, P.E., Cannon, J.G., et al., "Effect of vitamin E and eccentric exercise on selected biomarkers of oxidative stress in young and elderly men," *Free Radical Biology and Medicine*, 34: 1575–88, 2003.

Tengardy, R.P., "The role of vitamin E in the immune response and disease resistance," *Annals of the New York Academy of Science*, 587: 24–33, 1990.

Thompson, D., Williams, C., McGregor, S.J., et al., "Prolonged vitamin C supplementation and recovery from demanding exercise," *International Journal of Sport Nutrition and Exercise Metabolism*, 11: 466–81, 2001.

Urso, M.L., and Clarkson, P.M., "Oxidative stress, exercise, and antioxidant supplementation," *Toxicology*, 189: 41–54, 2003.

Chapter 12: How Muscles Work and Grow

Armstrong, R.B., "Influence of exercise training on O_2 delivery to skeletal muscle," IN: The Lung: Scientific Foundations, R.G. Crystal, J.B. West et al. (Eds.). New York: Raven Press, Ltd., 1991, pp. 1517–1524.

Biolo, G., Tipton, K.D., Klein, S., et al., "An abundant supply of amino acids enhances the metabolic effect of exercise on muscle protein," *American Journal of Physiology*, 273: E122–E119, 1997.

Bloom, W., and Fawcett, D.W., A Textbook of Histology. Philadelphia: W.B. Saunders, Co. 1975.

Brooks, G.A., Fahey, T.D., White, T.P., and Baldwin, K.M., Exercise Physiology: Human Bioenergetics and Its Applications, (3rd edition), Mayfield Publishing Co. Mountain View, CA, 2000.

Costill, D.L., Coyle, E.F., Fink, W.F., Lesmes, G.R., and Witzmann, F.A., "Adaptations in skeletal muscle following strength training," *Journal of Applied Physiology*, 46: 96–99, 1979.

Coyle, E.F., Feltner, M.E., Kautz, S.A., et al., "Physiological and biomechanical factors associated with elite endurance cycling performance," *Medicine and Science in Sports Exercise*, 23: 93–107, 1991.

Gollnick, P.D., and Hermansen, L., "Biochemical adaptations to exercise: anaerobic metabolism," IN: Exercise and Sport Sciences Reviews, Vol. 1. J.H. Wilmore (Ed.). New York: Academic Press, 1973, pp. 143.

Gonyea, W.J., Sales, D.G., Gonyea, F.B., and Mikesky, A., "Exercise induced increases in muscle fiber number," *Journal of Applied Physiology*, 55: 137–141, 1986.

Hermansen, L., Hultman, E., and Saltin, B., "Muscle glycogen during prolonged severe exercise," *Acta Physiologica Scandanavic*, 71: 129–139, 1967.

Holloszy, J.O., "Biochemical adaptations to exercise: aerobic metabolism," IN: Exercise and Sport Sciences Reviews, Vol. 1. J H. Wilmore (Ed.). New York: Academic Press, 1973, pp. 4471.

Ivy, J.L., "Exercise physiology and adaptations to training," IN: Handbook of Exercise in Diabetes. N. Ruberman (Ed.) American Diabetes Association, 2002, pp. 23–62.

Ivy, J.L., Withers, R.T., VanHandel, P.J., Elger, D.E., and Costill, D.L., "Muscle respiratory capacity and fiber type as determinants of the lactate threshold," *Journal of Applied Physiology*, 48: 523–527, 1980.

MacDougall, J.D., "Morphological changes in human skeletal muscle following strength training and immobilization," IN: Human Muscle Power. N.L. Jones, N. McCartney, A.J. McComas (Eds.). Champaign, IL: Human Kinetics, 1986, pp. 269–288.

MacDougall, J.D., Tuxen, D., Sale, D.G., Moroz, J.R., and Sutton, J.R., "Arterial blood pressure response to heavy resistance exercise," *Journal of Applied Physiology*, 58: 785–799, 1985.

Rowell, L.B., Human Circulation. Regulation During Physical Stress, New York: Oxford Press Inc., 1986.

Sale, D.L., "Influence of exercise and training on motor unit activation," IN: Exercise and Sport Sciences Reviews, Vol. 15. K.B. Pandolf (Ed.). New York: MacMillan. 1987, pp. 95–152.

Saltin, B., Henriksson, J., Nyaard, E., et al., "Fiber types and metabolic potentials of skeletal muscles in sedentary man and endurance runners." IN: The Marathon: Physiological, Medical, Epidemiological, and Psychological Studies, Annals of the New York Academy of Sciences, Vol. 301. P. Milvy (Ed.). NewYork, NY, 1977, pp. 3–29.

Saltin, B., and Rowell, L.B., "Functional adaptations to physical activity and inactivity," *Federation Proceedings*, 39: 1506–l513, 1980.

Schaible, T.F., and Scheur, J., "Cardiac adaptation to exercise," *Progress in Cardiovascular Disease*, 27: 297–324, 1985.

Wilmore, J.H., and Costill, D.L., Training for Sport and Activity. The Physiological Basis of the Conditioning Process, (3rd edition), Dubuque, IA: Wm. C. Brown Publishers, 1988.

Index

About the Authors

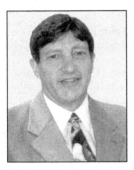

John Ivy is Chair and Margie Gurley Seay Centennial Professor in the Department of Kinesiology & Health Education at the University of Texas at Austin. He received his Ph.D. in Exercise Physiology from the University of Maryland and his postdoctoral training in physiology and biochemistry from Washington University School of Medicine. He has published over 150 research papers on the effects of nutrition on physical performance and exercise recovery. He is a Fellow and former Ambassador for the American College of Sports Medicine and Fellow in the American Academy of Kinesiology.

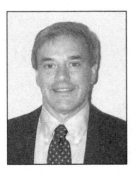

Robert Portman earned his Ph.D. in biochemistry from Virginia Tech. He has numerous scientific publications and has written and lectured extensively on the role of nutrition in improving exercise performance. Dr. Portman is head of research at PacificHealth Laboratories, a nutrition technology company that has pioneered in the development of innovative nutritional products to help athletes reach their potential.